BECOMING THE ROCKET SHAMAN

Lessons in Healing Chronic Illness, Emotional Pain, and Burnout When Nothing Else Works

"Simon Luthi's journey reminds us that the most resilient path is often the one that leads us home to ourselves. Say "Yes" to this profound invitation to redefine healing, leadership, and what it truly means to rise resilient."

—Dr. Taryn Marie Stejskal
#1 *Wall Street Journal* Bestselling Author,
Founder of the Resilience Leadership Institute

"Simon guides you to find a renewed outlook on life, through the inspiration of desperation."

—Ernesto Arguello
Social Innovator and Friend

"We never know when it's over—Simon's book reminds us to live fully, love fiercely, and care for your body, mind, and soul with intention."

—Sibylle Spühler-Moran
Fellow survivor, entrepreneur, and
former Mrs. Switzerland 2007

"With wisdom, vulnerability, and insight, Simon offers a path to true healing, especially for those who feel like they've tried everything. *Becoming the Rocket Shaman* is the kind of book that doesn't just offer hope. It restores it."

—Ashley Arguello
CEO of CanWe

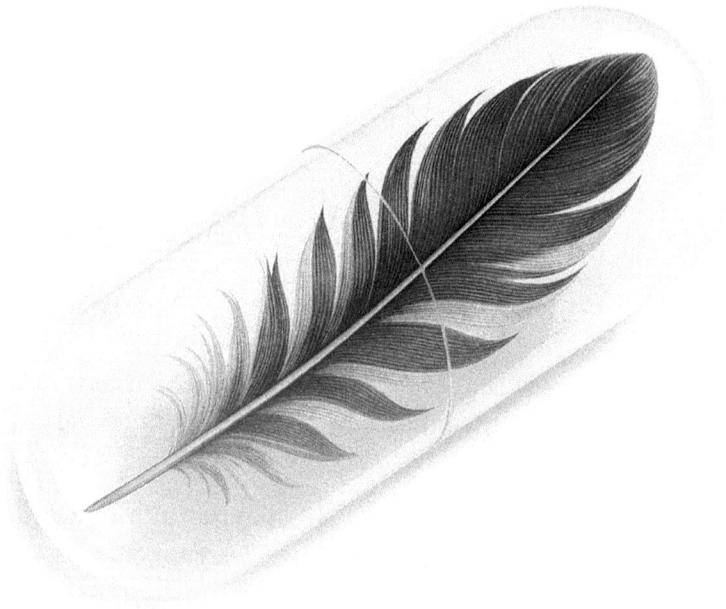

The Frequency That Changes Everything.[IP]
Words plant the seed. Music grows the forest.

What you're about to read will challenge, inspire, and awaken you. What you're about to hear will rewire your reality.

During my training as a sound engineer in the early '90s, my friend Jeff demonstrated something astonishing—he could influence the crowd's emotions with the turn of a knob. What I felt intuitively then is now proven: frequency vibrations—at levels humans can't hear—trigger mood-boosting chemicals like serotonin and dopamine, activating deep brain regions, and measurably reducing stress hormones.[1]

We don't merely listen to sound waves—our bodies absorb them.

While writing this book, my dormant passion for music awakened. I heard distinct energy in each chapter and felt compelled to transmute these sensations into song. From rock to high-vibe chill, each song reflects many moods and parts of the self. Each track corresponds to a chapter, energetically crafted to amplify the transformational power of learning, loving, and healing.

Please turn up the volume in your car before reading or dance in your kitchen after completing a chapter.

This album isn't just musical storytelling— it's engineered transformation.

During mastering, I wove specific frequencies throughout each track, including subsonic and harmonic layers that work below conscious awareness. You're not just hearing my journey—you're receiving a sonic transmission designed to regulate your nervous system and catalyze your transformation. Each track corresponds to a chapter, engineered to amplify its transformational power.

Reading this book without the frequency medicine is like taking half the prescription.

Music anchors memory. Sound rewires neural pathways. Together, they create change that neither can achieve alone. Cells react to vibration before words. The nervous system trusts frequency over logic. The soul recognizes its melody before releasing its story.

Don't leave your transformation incomplete.

Welcome to Becoming the Rocket Shaman. Let the words carry you, and the music elevate you to who you already are.

Unlock the Full Transmission
Your healing deserves to be heard.
To download the companion album,
Whispers From the Healing Road[IP],
visit https://bit.ly/TRSMusic
or scan the QR above.

BECOMING THE ROCKET SHAMAN

Lessons in Healing Chronic Illness, Emotional Pain, and Burnout When Nothing Else Works

Simon Lüthi

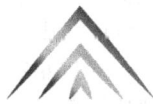

THE ROCKET SHAMAN
LEADERSHIP ACADEMY

Published by The Rocket Shaman Leadership Academy[IP]

Paperback ISBN: 978-1-965419-24-3
Hardcover ISBN: 978-1-965419-25-0
e-Book ISBN: 978-1-965419-26-7
Library of Congress Control Number: 2025918165

Available in paperback, hardcover, e-book, and audiobook.

This is a work of nonfiction.
Some names and identifying details may have been changed to protect the privacy of individuals.

Printed in the United States of America.

The superscript symbol IP listed throughout this book is known as the unique certification mark created and owned by Instant IP[IP]. Its use signifies that the corresponding expression (words, phrases, chart, graph, etc.) has been protected by Instant IP[IP] via smart contract. Instant IP[IP] is designed with the patented smart contract solution (US Patent: 11,928,748), which creates an immutable time-stamped first layer and fast layer identifying the moment in time an idea is filed on the blockchain. This solution can be used in defending intellectual property protection. Infringing upon the respective intellectual property, i.e., IP, is subject to and punishable in a court of law.

I dedicate this book to my late mother,
as without her serendipitous posthumous interventions
and divine interactions, this book would
never have been written.

CONTENTS

PRELAUNCH

THE GREAT UNRAVELING[IP]: CREATING SPACE TO LIVE IT UP

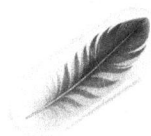

Can my body finish this bike ride? Three months have passed since being declared cancer-free. Today is the first of a thirteen-day, 1,000-kilometer cycling expedition. Starting through the Lavaux terraced vineyards—a UNESCO World Heritage Site where grapevines hug the shores of Lake Geneva, Switzerland—the path winds through a chain of Alpine foothills. After finishing at a medieval town on the Swiss side of Lake Constance, where three bodies of water merge, I will pass by streams and lakes so clean, I can see to the bottom. This excursion has been on my "new beginnings" list for over four years.

Having faced death multiple times, the idea of chasing a bucket list for the rest of my life feels oddly morbid to me. Even though it has taken me fifty-one years to reconcile my emotional differences with dying, I relish knowing that if I live only one more day, with a new opportunity opening to me every second, I have 86,400 opportunities to start anew. Adventure, like butterflies moving en masse, fluttering about a garden, is a lively feeling that I want to recreate over and over again.

Earlier today, I found my pace and rode through many villages, progressively more rural in the days ahead. This trip to

Switzerland is one to make peace with the country I left with bitterness in my 20s. It's funny how easy it is to blame a geographical location for things not working out the way we want, as if the land is at fault. Switzerland is guilty by association for my childhood disappointments and a midlife, post-divorce breakup with a woman I hoped would be my next serious partner. When I moved to the United States, I did so on the premise that I could never find true love or belonging. Returning all these years later, to do this ride alone, I trust I can heal the remaining scars I'm carrying.

As it happens, *Herzroute* is the official German name of the bike route. This translates to "Heart Route" in English. The Swiss people consider the Latin name of Switzerland, Helvetia, to personify the country as female. What better place to mend my unresolved past with women? It's kismet!

When I reached the top of the first hill this afternoon, one of many I will climb in the coming days, I stopped to look back upon the scenery and admired how far I had come. Turning around, smiling a bit out of breath, I tilted my head back slightly and put my hands on my hips. I leaned side to side, then front to back to stretch my spine. Turning around, I paused, staring in awe at the beauty in the distance; the hamlets I passed were now little white and orange clusters. I understood the breadth of the journey I had begun and blurted aloud, "Oh, shit. I can actually do this!" This sudden burst of faith acknowledged that I had accomplished a great deal that day. Turning to my bike I had laid down beside me, I bent down, then gripped the handlebars affirmatively. *I am ready. I want to keep going.* In the days ahead, I approach the ride as a moving meditation—briefly closing my eyes, then opening them, taking in the landscape as if I am seeing it for the first time.

On the fifth day, for no other reason than a strong feeling in my gut, I dedicated a particular stretch of the route to my father, who passed away a few years ago. An avid cyclist, he would have wanted to take a bike ride such as this with me.

At eighty years old, my father asked, "What could I have done to be a better parent?" He believed he hadn't done his best. As adults, my siblings and I had made this known to him, sharing our feelings about the pressure he had placed on us to be successful in our youth. We never thought Dad listened to us, nor did we ever believe we could meet his standards. Turns out we were wrong. By asking me what he could have done better, we came to a mutual understanding and put our differences to rest.

My father shared information I never would have known had he not confronted the past to build a relationship with me.

My father's parents sent him to live with his grandparents when they divorced. They assumed the role of guardians. His grandmother struggled with alcohol, and his grandfather exhibited a need to exert control over the household. My dad's future became a byproduct of his grandfather's authority. He was determined to make my father believe he would never make it as an architect, casting a shadow on his dreams. He demanded that my father attend college to become a teacher. Dad didn't argue because he learned that challenging others' beliefs, especially elders', is disrespectful.

While the role of a teacher is noble, he believed he certainly could have been in worse circumstances. Still, my father's story is a familiar narrative for many. His idea of success morphed into what he had perceived as values. He lived according to what the world deemed secure, adopted the doctrines of others rather than living on his terms, and unknowingly passed the pattern on to his children.

I became woven into a generational quilt that replaced inspiration and possibility with fear. I had to learn how to break the cycle by reframing my past.

Learning more about my father's upbringing allowed me to understand why he was insistent that stellar grades, money, and clout would keep his kids safe. Ironically, I discovered that the relentless pursuit of those goals was the principal contributor to the insecurities I developed in middle age.

Over time, my lack of confidence created behaviors that manifested as autoimmune disease and cancer. By opening up to me during that late stage of his life, Dad supported me in breaking the cycle within our family. The conversation between us opened a metaphorical door, releasing a variety of emotions that had been stagnant in my body. As a result, my father and I developed a deeper appreciation for our newly built relationship in the years before he passed.

All hidden secrets were gone; only truths remained. Neither of us made any excuses for our behavior. We liberated ourselves from a painful history.

As I ride on, recalling memories of the conversations we had before he took his last breath, I feel a release in processing my grief. I know his spirit is riding next to me.

On the sixth morning of the ride, I wake knowing that it is the day I will ask my spiritual home for forgiveness for running away. Without knowledge of when or where, I'll make peace with my past; I need to trust Spirit will direct me to the right place at the perfect moment. I request a spot where I can plant my bare feet on the ground, pray, and humbly ask to be pardoned. "Okay, Spirit, show me where I should hold this ritual today."

Storming out of Switzerland, I felt brash. I resented the culture because I hadn't gotten my way. I believed there was no apparent reason for me to repent, but holding my past in contempt was immature. The negative emotions in my body needed to be released to create space for future good; they no longer served me.

Just as my father wasn't to blame for how my life turned out, the country I grew up in wasn't to blame either. I am the only one responsible for my life.

As I ride up and down the hillsides, the vineyard land-scape remains in the distance. Pastoral lands dotted with cows become the scenery in the middle of the rural region of Emmental, home of the original Swiss cheese. Steadily, I make my way up a steep gravel road. Alternating stretches of warm, direct sunlight with pockets of lush, deep green forest, the landscape changes. The path provides necessary shade and a cool breeze once the unforgiving heat takes position overhead. With my hands gently on the handlebars, I relax and find comfort in the outdoors' natural ventilation. I feel my bike tug ever so slightly to the left. This is an indicator signaling that I have reached my destination for the forgiveness ritual.

I place my bike down and step through a nature-made door into the forest. As if God is calling, three tree stumps, two covered in moss, and one with a large, resting, white feather, appeared. "Son, this is the place. Here is your altar."

Cancer, the mystery illness, and all the moments that brought me to the bike ride. From unhealthy and dissatisfied, I evolved into someone filled with compassion. Now, my wish is to extend the love I felt in my earlier years, when I believed the universe was against me, and bring you on a journey of transformation that saved my life—that redeemed me.

I remove my shoes and socks, feel my feet hit the cool, woodsy ground, and topple into a silent meditation. A divine presence, with quiet curiosity, is there to greet me. Into the silence, I speak, "Can you please connect me with the people who will support my future life?"

"Yes." The resounding response travels through my body.

The voice reverberates from my forehead to my toes; specifically, who will arrive and when will only reveal itself at the appropriate time. Positive connections are being forged with the past, allowing more space to welcome revitalized relationships. I continue to pray for physical and emotional strength to make it through to the end of the ride.

The following day, my right knee feels like it's giving out. I pause intermittently to stretch and lessen the ache. Realizing I need assurance, I pose the same question to Spirit I asked the first day, "Can my body make it through to the end of this ride?"

Although sweat runs down my face, all doubt disappears. The challenges I've gone through to get here will not stop me from getting back on my bike. As I move toward the finish line, I block out the pain. "Can my body make it through to the end of this ride?" With a resounding "yes," all uncertainty is pushed aside. First, a whisper, the affirmation grows into a proclamation that I declare. I approach the finish line. Still admiring the landscape that surrounds me, I continue to ask myself the all-important question. My knee remains stiff and swollen.

In the moments I feel pressed against my limitations, I stare down the threshold of my endurance.

I speak affirmatively to the pain, release it, then pedal on.

On the 13th and final day of cycling the Herzroute, the flywheel releases one more time. I reach the top of the last hill and descend towards the finish line, approaching sea level as though I have conquered the summit of a glorious, snow-laced Alpine mountain.

I look out at the view of Lake Constance at the end of the Herzroute, and see the richness of my past in the glory of the majestic Alpine landscape.

How did I overlook its stunning beauty?

My body got me to the finish line, but Spirit transformed the entire view.

INTRODUCING THE ROCKET RESET[IP]: TRANSCENDING THE FEAR-BASED WORLD

I would never have considered writing a book if the call to do so hadn't come through on the very day of my mother's passing. While on Earth, Mom set aside her needs to care for others. When she transitioned, I knew she would be an active presence guiding my life. She sent many signs, checking in, and showing support.

> The term *transitioning* as a metaphor for dying originates from the idea of death as a passage or change from one state of existence to another, rather than an end. Rooted in numerous spiritual and philosophical traditions, this term reflects beliefs in an afterlife, reincarnation, or a journey to a different realm. It softens the finality of death, emphasizing continuity, transformation, and the idea that life "transitions" to a different form or phase. This concept is often used in more compassionate or spiritual discussions about death.

On the day Mom left Earth, she sent several remarkable people my way. Each of them expressed an interest in my story. Through many engaging conversations, I sensed my mother's nudge to write a book and responded with a resounding "yes!"

In the spring after I began my authorship journey, my home security camera captured a robin repeatedly flying with dominant force into the glass pane of my front door. In the coming days, the bird continued to appear. Toward the end of that week, I talked with my friend Rick about our shamanic work, specifically in helping people transition peacefully.

Unprompted by me, he began speaking about the symbolism of the robin. "They are messengers for the other side," he said. "They want to tell you, 'I'm still here. I'm looking after you, and I love you." When I told him about the robin that had come to my door, he advised me to acknowledge it. The robin returned the following morning. I went outside and called it by my mother's name. "Thank you for looking out for me. I love you." After hearing those words, the bird flew off and never returned. I understood it had finished its mission.

I want to assure you that if you remain open to possibilities, you may encounter more pleasant surprises than you realize. When I got sick, I realized that the unexpected, unpleasant events that caused me pain and suffering were invitations to live with purpose. I found my calling.

The Rocket Shaman[IP]

My brother, Valentin, is the person who first coined me The Rocket Shaman. He went through shamanic training long before I considered doing so. After I got sick, witnessing his work inspired me to explore ancient wisdom to heal. I studied and trained to become a Neo-Shaman.

Unlike traditional shamanism, Neo-Shamanism is more eclectic, often integrating elements from shamanic traditions worldwide. Neo-Shamanism adapts to the context of Western society. We don't live in remote areas. We have different stressors. I immediately embraced the blending of the modern and ancient worlds. After my shamanic initiation, my healing practice took off much faster than I, or anyone else, expected.

Valentin found the rapid growth of my practice amusing, given that I had been a skeptic of the healing arts. One evening, I overheard him speaking to a friend in his thick Swiss-German accent. "Simon didn't even vant anytzing to do vith spirituality seven years ago. Vonce he said yes, he took off like a rocket. He's Ze Rocket shaman." The name sounded uplifting. I embraced it seriously. Becoming Ze Rocket shaman propelled me into a new stratosphere in my life, challenging me to think beyond my current reality.

Rockets aren't only vessels of speed. They are constructed with resilient, lightweight materials built to withstand extreme conditions. Humans are no different, but we get weighed down, pulled in directions far from the life we choose. To be aerodynamic, we must go deep to excavate and release the heavy burdens holding us back and tune in to our inner knowing. That's where the work of a shaman comes in.

Throughout this book, I've included citations to honor both the wisdom keepers and scientists whose teachings and research have illuminated these practices—they deserve recognition, and their work adds depth to our understanding. While I deeply value their contributions, please remember that the most important voice here is yours. I invite you to approach everything in these pages with curiosity, questioning what doesn't resonate and trusting your own inner wisdom as your truest guide.

I use the word shaman in reverence to those who taught me. There are misinterpretations of shamanism and exploitation of Indigenous people by some Westerners. I uphold the integrity of what I've learned, using my gifts in a way that's authentic to who I am and respectful toward my teachers.

I need to be up front with you about who I am and the contrasting sides of myself. I'm not a guru, and I don't wear flowy linen clothes. My favorite things to wear are cotton T-shirts, jeans, and sneakers. I love to drink green juice and smudge my house by burning tree resins and herbs. On Friday evenings, while cooking dinner, I appreciate bourbon and listening to '70s rock. Crystals and mystical art fill my home. I spin pottery and use the imperfect pieces to hold scented wax candles. I still drive the Maserati that I bought as a corporate executive. I've been trying to sell it for years, but no one will buy it. Acknowledging all aspects of myself liberates me from fear—no more hiding. I hope you discover and embrace the different facets of your identity as you read. May you surprise yourself.

One of the most fun parts of my journey has been learning a new language. Throughout this book, I explain the meanings and origins of words that may seem unusual to you. I hope that the words in this book, many of which are derived from ancient cultures, inspire you to rethink how you talk about your life.

Many teachings that were passed down to me by my teachers, among them, the Q'ero People. I will pass what they taught me to you at the beginning of each section of this book—Learn, Love, Heal, and Becoming The Rocket Shaman.

Why I Wrote This Book

Why am I still here when so many are not? That question found perhaps its sharpest edge in the passing of my friend, Amber Kelleher-Andrews. Although we only knew each other for a short amount of time, it was clear to me that she was a radiant bridge between people, between worlds. Her presence lit up every room. Her love was boundless. When she transitioned, it broke something open in me. A grief that turned into fuel. A love that demanded action. I kept asking: *Why am I here and she's not? Why do so many people die young?*

This question haunted me, as I know it haunts you when death steals someone too soon. In this single, aching question lies the entire mystery of human existence. The question that has tormented hearts for centuries, that wakes us at 3 a.m., that no philosophy can fully answer.

When Amber died, something ignited in me; the same fire that sparks in all of us when death comes too early, too cruel. It's more than remembrance. More than honoring. It's a fierce, urgent calling that says: *Live. Now. Fully. Make it matter.*

This book is that calling made visible. It's not just about leaving a legacy; it's about transforming our pain into purpose, our questions into action, our brief time here into something that lights the way for others. I didn't write this book to impress you. I wrote it because I had to survive. Because I was dying—physically, emotionally, energetically—and I needed to find a way back to life. My breakdowns became my initiations. Chronic illness, divorce, and spiritual disconnection stripped me bare. And yet, they also revealed something ancient: that healing isn't just about getting better. It's about remembering who we were before the world told us to forget. Because maybe that's the answer to the unanswerable question: We're here to live so fully that our light continues long after we're gone.

One evening while crafting this book, Spirit spoke to me during the Human Oracle Card Ritual[IP] with a friend (I share the ritual in Chapter 2). I asked, *"Where should I share the messages in this book?"* The answer came quickly: *"Look to the illogical spaces."*

For thirty years as a corporate strategist and executive, I relied on what was "logical." When my health collapsed, my definition of logic changed. Some of the most highly trained doctors in the US couldn't diagnose my autoimmune disease. In searching for answers, I uncovered knowledge outside the healthcare system and found safe, effective ways to treat my illness. Knowing death could have been my outcome—and living for years without remembering what "healthy" felt like—drives me to share what I've learned.

I embrace both modern medicine and alternative healing, placing greater emphasis on energy work, food as medicine, and healthy habits. My goal is to stay far from hospitals, yet I acknowledge doctors have saved my life and mended my broken bones. All aspects of healthcare have value, but I share the frustration of many with an industry that fails to diagnose and support patients fully.

Being alive is a privilege. Tomorrow is never guaranteed. My long and healthy life isn't measured in years or hours, but in the strength to rise into a higher version of myself.

How to Approach This Book

Self-discovery is personal. You will find relatable messages in this book to inspire your path to a long and healthy life, but your path is uniquely yours.

While I honor those who originated and inspired the rituals and teachings shared here, the true expert is you. As you turn these pages, I encourage you to think independently.

Translating hardship into healing was often messy. My emotions swung from anger to bliss, shifting like sudden island weather. At my lowest, I wondered if the happiest days of my life were already behind me. It took nearly fifty years to unravel the fear-based messages I had internalized. I invite you to see that it is never too late to change. Consistency matters more than speed. I won't pretend your entire life will transform overnight, but even one small step in a new direction can spark progress and satisfaction.

Each section begins with a shamanic lesson, followed by a Story from my Healing Table and an essay. Sharing my stories is an invitation for you to craft your own narrative—one that lifts you higher. At the end of every chapter, you can move through the Reader Reflections, Actionable Insights, and a Spirited Act of Authenticity[IP]—a ritual you can practice at home.

Take what resonates and return as often as needed to reset any part of your life. Use this book as a companion, a non-judgmental space that believes no wound is too shallow or deep.

If you feel trapped in a recurring dream, unable to find your way home, this book is for you. Nothing in these pages is a quick fix or a guaranteed cure, nor should it replace professional treatment. Instead, it is a call to ask yourself what living a long and healthy life means to you. Imagine it. Activate it. Begin shaping the vision you choose for yourself.

With Gratitude

I write this book from my soul to yours. I share my experiences from a deep and vulnerable place to create a connection with you. Your experience is worthy of attention. I promise that once you understand them, you can find meaning and purpose when you look back and fly onward and upward as you welcome healing as a blissful and necessary part of being human. Thank you for being here with me. If there's anything I want you to take away from this book, it's that if I can heal myself, you can too.[IP]

So here we are, you and I. On this page. At this moment. In the middle of remembering. Let this book be your invitation. Let this be the moment your soul wakes up. You are still here because you are needed. Because we are in a time of great forgetting, and even greater remembering. Because the world is breaking open. And because now more than ever, we need people willing to rise from the fire and carry the medicine of their lived truth. And the world is waiting for your medicine. Because if you're holding this book, there's a reason. Because healing is no longer a luxury—it's a necessity.[IP] Because your pain, your story, your awakening—they matter. They are needed.

Ready? Great, then let's begin!

READER REFLECTION: THE GREAT UNRAVELING OF YOUR LIFE STARTS NOW

What emotional, mental, physical, and spiritual parts would you like to unpack?

What's good about staying the same? What's good about change?

Spirited Act of Authenticity: Create Your New Beginnings List[IP]

New beginnings can open up space for growth, healing, and creativity. Here's a simple guide to help you craft your own New Beginnings List and start living life with intention.

Reflect on Your Current Space

- Take a moment to pause and journal where you are in life right now—emotionally, mentally, physically, and spiritually.
- Ask yourself: *What areas of my life feel stagnant or need renewal?*
- Jot down any emotions, thoughts, or situations that come to mind as you reflect.

Let Go of the Past

- Release what no longer serves you. Think about the things you've been holding onto that prevent new experiences from entering your life.
- Write down at least one habit, belief, or situation you're ready to release.

Dream Boldly

- Allow yourself to dream without limits. What experiences, adventures, or personal transformations do you want to invite into your life?
- Add these dreams to your New Beginnings List to create a fresh space for joy, fulfillment, and growth.

Accept the Present Moment and Align It with Your Yes

- Embrace the idea that your life is constantly unfolding. Saying "yes" to what is happening now opens the door for more opportunities to flow into your life. Allow yourself to say, "A yes to my circumstances is a yes to seeing possibilities." We neglect to see the gifts and lessons in our experiences by denying, fighting, or resisting our present.

- Commit to being fully present and taking small, consistent actions toward the new beginnings you've listed. List three actions you can take toward making your list a reality.

Honor the Cycles of Time

- Just as the circular cross in shamanism symbolizes non-linearity, remember that time is non-linear. Trust that the past, present, and future are interconnected, and your new beginnings can heal and shape all parts of your life. Like me writing this book, they can appear unexpectedly at any time.

- Keep your list dynamic—allow it to evolve with you as you grow and change.

Revisit and Update

- Regularly revisit your New Beginnings List.
  - o What have you accomplished?
  - o What needs to be adjusted?
  - o What new desires have come up?

Use this list as a living document supporting your journey to becoming your truest self. Feel free to document on the following pages or create your own journal.

Sacred Scribbles[IP] (Use these pages as a portal for decoding visions, tracking soul whispers, or just letting the ink remember what your heart already knows.)

PART 1. LEARN

BUILD YOUR ROCKET

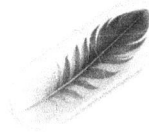

Before the world becomes one, before the people become one, before your beliefs become one, people will go crazy. But not until you understand that God is in a breath, in all that breathes, then it will become one. One faith.

—Grandmother Rita Pitka Blumenstein (Yup'ik Elder)

Western societies are facing deep challenges—from social upheaval and workplace stress to rising chronic illness and a growing mental health crisis. Many Indigenous people see this moment not only as a time of crisis but as an opportunity to share their wisdom and traditions.[2] From their perspective, the West is in the midst of a collective existential struggle, one that endangers both human well-being and the health of the planet. Within these challenges are possibilities for renewal and a more balanced way of living.

The story of the Q'ero people is one of resilience, prophecy, and preservation of ancient wisdom.[3] The descendants of the Inca live in the remote villages of the Peruvian Andes, where the landscape is as harsh as it is breathtaking. These high-altitude villages, tucked among jagged peaks and lush valleys, are so isolated that only those who've endured years of hardship can thrive there. In the 16th century, their journey began during the Spanish conquest of the Inca Empire. Among the Q'ero people are spiritual practitioners known as paqos, who have preserved and transmitted the ancient wisdom traditions. As the conquerors advanced, bringing destruction and disease, the Q'ero people sought refuge high in the Andes, away from the violent upheaval below. Their journey was not just a flight for survival; it was a conscious decision to protect their sacred traditions and the spiritual wisdom of their ancestors.

Today, nestled in the rugged mountains at altitudes exceeding 14,000 feet, the Q'ero people, including their paqos, have found sanctuary. The air is thin and sharp, every breath a reminder of their resilience. The wind howls through the valleys, the chill of the early mornings bites into the skin, and the warmth of the sun during the day feels like a precious gift. In this remote place, they preserve their traditions, their language, and their way of life. It's a life intimately connected to the natural world—the towering peaks, the rushing streams, the vibrant fields of quinoa and potatoes—all of which serve as their spiritual allies. Their existence, built on a deep reverence for the Earth and its cycles, remains virtually untouched by modern society.

The Q'ero prophecies are passed down through generations. These prophecies are more than predictions. They are a guide for navigating both personal and collective evolution. One significant prediction speaks of the coming of a new era—a time when the ice-capped mountains will melt. For the paqo, changes in the natural world are far from random; they are signs that the prophecy is nearing fulfillment.

As the prophecy predicted, in recent decades, the glaciers that once encircled their high-altitude homes have receded. The vast ice fields, which once seemed eternal, now lie scattered with jagged rocks and exposed earth. The Q'ero do not see this solely because of climate change. They see the melting glaciers as part of a greater spiritual unfolding—wisdom that the land held for a long time is awakening. It is a cosmic event that marks the return of sacred knowledge to the world during a time of crisis. The Q'ero paqos' descent from the mountains is a divine mandate to bring their teachings to the modern world, where the need for healing and renewal is greatest.

Traveling to the West is not a simple journey for these paqos. The world they are entering is unfamiliar, filled with distractions and dissonance. Their arrival, though welcomed by many, is fraught with challenges. Much of the modern world has lost touch with the spiritual wisdom that the Q'ero people carry. There is a tension between ancient ways and modern sensibilities, and the paqos must navigate a world that often views their rituals and teachings with skepticism. Their task is to remind us of what we've forgotten, helping us to unlearn the fear-based narratives that disconnect us from our true selves and the Earth. Despite these challenges, they persist. For the Q'ero paqo, this is a sacred journey of restoring harmony between humanity and the Earth.

The teachings of the Q'ero people invite us to listen deeply as we reflect on them. In a world filled with noise and distraction, the Q'ero offer a pathway to reawaken the inner voice that guides us toward healing and self-awareness. Their teachings remind us we can live intentionally, align our actions with nature's rhythms, and find hope amid contemporary crises. They ask us to remember that wisdom is not something to be found externally; it is something we carry within, waiting to be awakened.

STORY FROM THE HEALING TABLE: UNLEARNING BELIEFS THAT HOLD YOU BACK

When we are born, we are in a natural state of authenticity. Fresh out of the womb, bellowing, a baby is unafraid to ask the world to meet its needs. Being newly born is a symbol of purity and potential for growth. As we age, our identities are prone to becoming stunted by external influences.

The fear-based world comprises bad information and false conditioning that affect our actions and ultimately mold our relationship with ourselves and others. In our daily practice, this can look like unconsciously adding excess sugar into our diet or obsessively comparing ourselves with others on social media, creating addictions and cravings for more of what is unhealthy. Our behaviors are driven by the rapid influx of information in the form of abbreviated ideas, beliefs, and opinions. This makes it difficult to know if we are thinking for ourselves.

Bad information is anything we adopt as ours without thinking it through. False conditioning refers to the "shoulds" of life. For many people, the fear-based world subtly seeps through the fractures of our hearts first, carving out canyons of self-doubt and insecurities. This impelled my actions, shaping my existence upon a father's prescribed role, an executive's leadership tenets, and a man's appearance.

We must confront the fear-based reality to transform it. A reality where wars rage, individuals hurt others, and uncontrollable disasters, such as hurricanes, breed fear. Distancing from the fear-based world isn't about denying it. It is about creating powerful shifts in ourselves by translating tragedy into learning and growth. Messages hidden within illness and disease, existential guideposts[IP] I call them, urge us to stop and correct our path. As we redirect and evolve, the new course of our lives is filled with learning.

4

Existential guideposts can bring us closer to authenticity, purpose, healing, and our relationship with the things we can see and not see. When we start seeing them as neutral instead of positive or negative, we can use them to transform how we live our days.

John, a stressed-out sixty-three-year-old, blue-collar worker and former Baptist, came to see me, expressing that he often had "weird feelings" that he described as premonitions. The sensations told him that something horrible was about to happen or someone terrible was going to show up in his life. He wanted to understand why he couldn't sleep. On the nights he did sleep, he was plagued with violent night terrors. The constant grinding of his teeth was causing muscle tension in his neck and shoulders. His religious background was often in the foreground of his thoughts as he pictured the judgment and ridicule he faced as a member of his church. He said he was taught to believe that God is a force waiting for him to screw up. Though he now deemed the information as untrue, he found it hard to submit to deeper spiritual pursuits.

John appeared to be a regular, American guy, dedicated to his career and family, riding a Harley on the weekends, and otherwise going through life on autopilot: work – eat – sleep – repeat. He kept his fears hidden behind a smile to ensure others remained undisturbed by him. Coming to see me was John's way of practicing the act of letting go. The predictions he made were his way of maintaining his old way of operating under his religion, scaring himself into falling in line with religious dogma.

Letting go is the conscious release of emotional attachment to past experiences, relationships, or outcomes, allowing oneself to move forward without being burdened by previous fears, hurts, or regrets. This process often involves acceptance, forgiveness, and the willingness to embrace uncertainty, making space for personal growth and new possibilities. As described by psychologist Carl Rogers, "The curious paradox is that when I accept myself just as I am, then I can change," highlighting that letting go often starts with accepting the present reality rather than resisting it.

As John traveled through life, he gained menacing spiritual hitchhikers—the kind that hold you up at gunpoint and steal your money after you trustingly offer them a ride. The trauma ruminated in his head as if they were driving while he was duct-taped to the passenger's seat. Though he thought the source of his pain was in his mind, during our work together, I quietly identified the vagrants' presence in his solar plexus, the area just above the belly button. The pressure was like a boulder sitting on his chest, tethering him to his past. This is what unrecognized existential guideposts can feel like. They accumulate, begging you to see their pain and confront it.

What followed was spiritual surgery of the gut, carried out over several energy-healing sessions. John's burdens became teachers, telling us where they were located in his body and asking to be freed from exile.

In John's case, a "**spiritual hitchhiker,**" or "energetic vampire," refers to an energy or entity that attaches itself to someone's spiritual journey, draining or influencing them negatively. It's believed in some spiritual traditions that such energies latch onto a person, especially when they are emotionally vulnerable or unprotected. This presence can create a range of blockages or distress, from brain fog to panic attacks, hindering spiritual progress and well-being, emphasizing the need for boundaries and awareness when exploring spiritual practices.

Each time John rose from my table, he spoke of feeling lighter, peaceful, beyond measure. His sleep improved, and he began having dreams instead of nightmares. One morning, he shared that he woke up laughing—a first in decades.

The hitchhikers exited his vehicle one by one, their influence dissolving as his energy shifted. John regained possession of the wheel. No longer a hostage to the rules that hurt him, he transmuted bad information and false conditioning into signals that helped him redirect his thoughts and actions. He resumed the same schedule and routine. He became more present, shifting from numb to enthusiastic and appreciative of the small things.

While we learn valuable lessons from others, I believe adopting doctrines that are not intrinsically our own is unhealthy. Carrying on in this way made me sick. Maybe it's gotten to you, too. If it has, I trust you will find freedom in the process to let it go like John did. You don't have to stop attending church services or change the way you vote. The important thing is that everything you do becomes aligned with the inner knowing that you are on the right path.

Nature Never Forgets

Between the ages of 24 months and five, children engage with the wondrous, conscious awareness of the ability to ask questions.[4] With persistent curiosity, toddlers often inquire, "Why?" repeatedly until they get a satisfying answer. Rather than dismissing the question by responding, "Because I said so," what if we observed this as a developmental stage in the child's learning? Acknowledge their need to understand. Ponder the answer. Engage them in exploring, "Why?" It may be that when you were a child, no one engaged in finding the answers, either. In many ways, adults are like children—still trying to find answers to many open-ended questions. With presence, learning, and extreme patience, they arrive.

Abstaining from inner wonder, as children, we are susceptible to bad information that conditions a false identity. In the process, intuition becomes confused with scarcity and fright, bred from hearing and believing everything around us, especially what we should fear. Focusing on what other people think, do, say, and feel, we lose sight of our true nature.

Self-exploration helps extract personal values and belief systems that feed a life lived on purpose. I invite you to ask questions again to learn and unlearn everything you need to know about who you are and transcend a fear-based world filled with bad information and false conditioning. You can become a well-informed luminary of your life by harnessing your intuition and using existential guideposts to your advantage.

After the last session I had with John, he reported that his sleep and outlook on life continued to improve. As a result, the mundane life he was leading became rich with gratitude for his family, his career, and the subtle joys nature provides. "Simon, I have a question. If nature always goes back to a state of order, and a cut heals, and the skin returns to normal, if lizard tails can grow back or a burned forest restores itself, why is it that evil, chaos, and discord seem to prevail? Why doesn't order, peace, and harmony?"

It's a profound question, isn't it? Why, if nature always returns to harmony—if cuts heal, forests regrow, and lizard tails regenerate—does it so often feel like chaos, suffering, and darkness are winning?

Initially, I didn't have an answer for John, but the question stayed with me. It echoed through my healing journey, through autoimmune disease, cancer, heartbreak, spiritual awakening, and became the seed of this book.

Nature never forgets how to heal.[IP] It doesn't resist life. Nature follows universal laws. Humans interrupt them. By learning through our experiences, our capacity to disconnect from what doesn't serve us increases because we know it's not ours to carry. We sync with nature's rhythm, our divine make-up, and everything changes for the better.

When evil, pain, or disorder seems to dominate, it's not the failure of the universe; it's a sign that we've strayed from our original design. The suffering isn't meaningless. It's a wake-up call—a sacred nudge to remember, return, and realign.

1

THE CONCEPTION OF IDENTITY: THE REBIRTH OF YOUR AUTHENTIC SELF

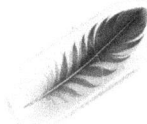

I n my late 40s, work consumed me. I tried hard to fulfill the joy-draining prophecy that life falls into place when we reach certain financial milestones. When I failed to get recognition for a project I led at work, I thought I wasn't doing enough. When I got promoted, I still thought I wasn't doing enough. No matter what I earned, it wasn't enough. *I* wasn't enough. The solution to my low self-worth was funneling all my time and energy into getting to the top of the corporate ladder. There was a lack of honesty in who I was, not because I intentionally lied or faked it; it was a fear of external rejection that kept me under constant pressure. I believed that if I didn't provide my family with a big house, new cars, and college tuition, I would be a failure.

As we walk toward the adult version of ourselves, too often we allow the world to coerce us into how we show up in life. A child-like voice whispers in our ears, wondering when we will pause, turn around, and really listen to them, questioning: "Do you know who you truly are?" I was gifted with unpleasant surprises from birth, forcing me to face my inner and outer adversaries, scaring me into living a life I wasn't actively choosing.

What I first discovered is that the core of my suffering was allowing my life to be built for me instead of by me. After that, I embraced that I could change anything I didn't like, approaching each moment as a chance to redirect my destiny through the lens of what I could learn from any given situation.

Between the ages of three and five, children study others intensively. They begin grouping people by their physical attributes, wondering where they fit in, and asking questions about their differences. At this point in childhood, the false information and stereotypes compound. What about before we meet the world or even begin developing in our mother's womb?

Both subtle and startling moments can have the biggest impact on our identity. In my case, I discovered some things that affected who I would become happened before conception. It wasn't until my mother lay on her deathbed that she explained to me why one of my grandmothers never treated me lovingly. This revelation made me realize that the person I had defined as myself for nearly fifty years was a fabrication shaped by the perceptions and projections of others.

Building the False Self

After my twin siblings were born and before I was in utero, my mother nearly bled to death from a tubal pregnancy that did not come to fruition. With only one fallopian tube, when she became pregnant with me, her life was threatened again. My parents' choice involved trying for a fourth child, despite my mother's past experiences and potential future dangers. This time, the baby, later known as me, would survive, and thankfully, so would my mother. From birth, core aspects of my identity were already in motion due to the circumstances surrounding conception, which endangered my mother.

As early as I can remember, there was always tension between my father's mother, Grandma Ingrid, and me. On the other hand, my mother's mother, Grandma Olivia, nurtured me and considered me a miracle after all my mother had endured. She even said I was a savior to her because my birth brought her happiness after her husband, my grandfather, passed away.

My mother shared that Grandma Ingrid challenged my mother's enthusiasm for her pregnancy. "You were denied a child once before. Why would you consider risking your life again?" She thought my parents were irresponsible for going forward with the pregnancy. Though she disliked church, she declared that God made it clear they ought not attempt to have another infant. I'm sure she was worried about losing her daughter-in-law, afraid her son would be left without his wife. Still, her fear made an already scary situation even harder for my parents.

I was born into polarizing circumstances when it came to the relationship with my grandmothers. To Grandmother Ingrid, I was not a risk worth taking. To Grandmother Olivia, I was a miracle baby. Grandma Olivia had just lost my grandfather. My birth was a symbol of new life that comforted her.

Practicing healing arts for several years, it wasn't until I was fifty-four, when my mother offered me the truth about my grandmother's feelings about my conception, that I could wholly understand how early my false identity began.

During childhood, I could not logically comprehend these issues.

I felt internal friction from a persistent unanswered question that I kept to myself until that conversation with my mother.

Why didn't Grandma Ingrid love me?

My mother's answer? "Because you were born against her will."

While this might seem unfair, the answer set me free. Knowing the history, I now knew that it wasn't my fault. I didn't want to be a death threat to my mother or the messiah in the wake of my grandfather's death. I wanted a chance to be myself. The stamp of the rescuer eventually led to me showing up as a "fixer" in my intimate relationships, forming a belief that I could buy myself love. Being seen as a burden gradually shaped a belief that something was inherently wrong with me, which led to years of bullying, low self-worth, and constant rejection by girls.

Early on, I decided that love was conditional. Knowing that, I internalized that I had to earn love. I never thought that love would come into my life by being myself. It seemed important to please people and fulfill their needs to gain their admiration. I modified my persona for the audience or the individual. Instead of deep love, I was unknowingly seeking validation. I stayed quiet, did what I was told, and became increasingly isolated and insecure.

Despite knowing I hated spending time with Grandma Ingrid, as the youngest of four by six years, when my parents needed a vacation, they shipped me off to stay with her. She lived in the same house her whole life. When I visited, she forced me to nap on horse-hair mattresses dating back to when my dad was born. It was one of her many relics; it's no wonder the bed was so uncomfortable. Its musty scent was overpowering. When I wasn't on the mattress, she would put me in front of the television.

On one of my visits, I watched an episode of the bizarre 1968 film Chitty Chitty Bang Bang.[5] Sitting in front of the television on the floor, I recall watching "The Child Catcher Scene." A creepy, pale-faced stranger wearing a top hat decorated with fake red and yellow flowers was jingling a bell, luring the children to follow him by dangling a bouquet of lollipops in his hand. "Come along, kiddie winkies," he said as he danced toward his horse and carriage. The children, entranced by promises of free ice cream and lollipops, follow him. Arriving at what looks like a circus tent, he lures them inside. Once they enter, he secures the entrance, revealing the tent's deception. Watching them being kidnapped and trapped in a cage reminded me of how I felt at Grandma Ingrid's house. Looking back on it now, it's an appropriate metaphor: A fear-based world entices us with empty promises only to fool us into thinking material things make love and happiness more attainable.

On another occasion, when Ingrid left me in the living room to watch television by myself, she turned on a show I had no interest in watching and left the room. Naturally, I got up to change the channel and chose to watch soccer. Returning to the room, she began screaming at me for touching the television. "This is my house," I recall these words and the homesickness I felt at that moment. With the television silenced, she departed, leaving me in solitude for the evening, devoid of both toys and companionship.

These seemingly small moments left me feeling abandoned, lonely, and sure that I had done something wrong by solely existing. Before I turned five, my false identity began insulating my internal walls. Little did I realize that the under-construction castle was surrounded by a moat infested with illness. Brick by heavy brick, layers of false narratives based on subtly damaging experiences were nailed together, framing who I thought I was.

Feelings similar to those with Grandma Ingrid were present in memories with other family members. I grew afraid to make a mistake because that is what I felt like simply by being there. Not only that, but the dynamic at home became unpredictable, especially between my father, my siblings, and me. He often yelled at us for making mistakes.

Dad taught physics and kept a toolbox of different gadgets. One of them was a battery tester. In those days, the batteries were square, with two latches connected to whatever device they were powering. Finding the tester, I thought it looked like a night light because it had a light bulb attached to it that would illuminate to signal that the battery was full. Living in Switzerland, our power was 220 volts, and the tester was nine volts, but I was five years old and did not remotely understand science.

Excitedly, I ran to my room to plug in the new night-light. When I plugged it into the socket, a loud "Boom!" sounded. The power went out in the house. Immediately, I feared my dad would come screaming. To avoid him, I ran and hid under the bed, hoping he wouldn't realize I was the one who caused the problem. I can't recall exactly how long I stayed there, but I remember it felt like hours. Eventually, my sister found me. "Hey, come out of there," she said. I resisted, telling her I was worried I would get beaten. "He's not mad, Simon," she said softly.

After my sister convinced me to slide out from under the bed, Dad explained to me that he was worried I could've electrocuted myself. To my surprise, his words were tender and loving toward me. Dad was unpredictable. He was likely experiencing the stress of everyday life, working to provide for us. The internal fear I felt when the lightbulb burst was a reaction from prior experiences when Dad got mad. When the nightlight blew up in my face, the first thing that alerted my brain was that I was the cause of everything that went wrong. I believed that I would be scolded and left alone as punishment, so hiding under the bed would temporarily keep me from being blamed for, once again, screwing up.

The story of who I was prior to being born created a kid who considered himself a burden. Thus began the hurtful words I would repeatedly tell myself. Looking back, hiding under the bed after the house went dark was the moment I started storing my emotions in places that felt safe. Along my journey, I have discovered that minor blips of memories and scenes from our lives can reveal a great deal about who we are.

Sharing these moments is not to encourage living in the past. My hope is that you feel empowered to draft a new narrative of your life, create renewed associations with history, and find grace for others. We can rewrite our version of the past to serve our higher self—the one who is loved and belongs without doing a thing.

The Impact of Authentic Living

Authentic living has a profound impact on our health and longevity. By shedding the stress and emotional weight of trying to satisfy a fear-based world, we reduce the physical toll that stress takes on our bodies. Extensive research across fields like cardiology, immunology, and behavioral science confirms that chronic stress is a significant risk factor for conditions ranging from cardiovascular disease to autoimmune disorders. Studies from Harvard, the CDC's ACE study, and major medical journals point to the clear physiological link between prolonged stress exposure and disease development.[6] When we live authentically, we cultivate an inner peace that promotes physical, mental, and emotional well-being.

- **Reduced stress:** Authentic living reduces the stress that comes from trying to meet external expectations. We stop trying to fit into societal boxes and instead, embrace the freedom of being ourselves.

- **Improved health:** The reduction of stress allows our bodies to heal and function optimally. With less anxiety and emotional turmoil, we experience better sleep, a stronger immune system, and more energy.

- **Longevity:** Decades of research show that people who live with a clear sense of purpose and inner alignment not only report greater well-being, but they live longer, healthier lives. Purpose is associated with lower inflammation, stronger immunity, and a significantly reduced risk of disease and early death. When we are connected to our true purpose and living authentically, we experience greater overall satisfaction with life, which contributes to long-term health.

Wake-Up Calls and Remembering

Every moment I denied myself the chance to hear what was being asked of me spiritually, the time and energy I spent living out of congruence with my authentic self stood between a false identity and what I now know to be me in my most authentic form. Like the scene in The Lion King where Mufasa comes down from the heavens to tell his son Simba, "Remember who you are," I believe many of us have forgotten that we are more than what we have become.[7]

If I hadn't become seriously ill three times in two years, I would have considered myself lucky to have overcome the symptoms of a mystery sickness. I would only have gone as deep as the shallow end would permit. With a cancer diagnosis, I was pushed into treacherous waters, forced to tread for my life, only to struggle catching my breath with every emotional riptide attempting to pull me under.

Eventually, I understood that if I remained committed to the process of determining what was making me sick, I could embrace the small child begging to notice him. By tending to my inner adolescence, I experienced the joy of understanding the core of my purpose, the being that defines how I now courageously live.

READER REFLECTION: THE FORMATION OF YOUR IDENTITY BEFORE CONCEPTION

Now is a time to reset the internal workings of your health by understanding your past, so that you can heal yourself emotionally, mentally, physically, and spiritually. An effective pathway to release the experiences you have attempted to forget is to adjust your perspective, renew your priorities, and learn from what has been traumatic, harmful, or seemingly useless. At the intersection of authenticity and purpose, you will transcend fear, angst, and unease and discover the total capacity of your existence. By circling back in time to make sense of the past, you will find out who you genuinely are.

What expectations do you believe were placed on your existence before you were born?

How have those expectations impacted how you show up emotionally, mentally, physically, and spiritually?

Imagine yourself free from the expectations of others. How do you see yourself showing up emotionally, mentally, physically, and spiritually?

ACTIONABLE INSIGHTS TO HEAL ACROSS FOUR DIMENSIONS OF HEALTH

Emotional

Releasing the need for external validation and embracing your true identity aids in experiencing deeper self-love and emotional freedom.

Mental

Challenging and reframing limiting beliefs from childhood can empower you by shifting into a clearer, more resilient mindset.

Physical

Identifying how unresolved emotions manifest in your body supports you in taking the right actions to restore balance and improve your overall well-being.

Spiritual

Aligning your actions with your inner truth leads to the ability to create a life filled with purpose and fulfillment.

SPIRITED ACT OF AUTHENTICITY: HOW TO ESTABLISH A SACRED SPACE INSIDE BY CREATING A PERSONAL ALTAR

As I was moving through my spiritual awakening, I instinctively started to sit in a comfy area of my home to meditate and calm my nervous system. This became my safe space to light a candle and reflect on my life. A lot of intuitive "aha" moments have started here. Some were more mundane, others profound. As you start with me on this journey toward your healing, I invite you to create a dedicated space in your home to set up your altar.

- The space should be quiet and allow you to escape the noise and business of life—a space dedicated just for you.

- It could be a spare bedroom that you could convert, a quiet area in your living room, or an attic waiting to be transformed.

- You want a piece of furniture that has special meaning or good energy. I used an old teak "v-shaped" chest that I found at an antique shop. You could also use an existing side table or refurbish a sideboard from a thrift store. It's important to have a vision of the feeling you want to create.

- I'd also suggest a cozy pillow or chair to sit comfortably for 30 minutes each day.

- You might find some additional inspiration online.

- If you have children or live with someone, ask them to respect this space as your own and not touch anything in it. This isn't meant to be overly religious or rigid. It's a way for you to retreat and focus either at the beginning or the end of your day, and it can be set up with little effort.

- Other items to consider: Use your imagination, but I suggest you don't forgo a candle and something to clear the energy daily. You can use traditional white sage or palo santo, or there are lavender/sage sprays with natural essential oils that you can buy at local organic food stores. I'll talk more about smudging and energy clearing in Chapter 4.

- I have picked up some special crystals and rocks along the way, which have special meanings. Some people feel connected to a cross, so that is fine to use as well. Some other people like to pray and meditate with a rosary. In my practice, I also use beautiful feathers that were gifted to me from the animal kingdom. (*Important*: Please check your local laws, as it is illegal to possess feathers from most native and migratory birds. Turkey feathers are a good alternative and readily available in most reputable crystal and metaphysical stores.)

- Most importantly, have fun with this. You will see the benefits of this as you move through the other rituals in this book.

If you don't have a dedicated space at home, you can create a peaceful environment by finding a place in nature. During my spiritual awakening, I discovered that being outdoors, even in a city park or a quiet spot on open land, was just as effective as any space at home. Whether it's a bench under a tree, a hidden corner of a park, or an open field you can revisit, nature offers a perfect sanctuary for reflection and calming your nervous system.

You don't need much—just a quiet spot to sit with intention. Bring a small blanket or cushion, or even just sit on the grass. If you are an avid traveler like me or live a more nomadic lifestyle, you can create a traveling altar. Bring a candle, incense, or a favorite object, or you can forgo bringing items with you and allow the natural environment to be grounding on its own. Focus on the sound of the wind, the feel of the earth, and the quiet that surrounds you.

Try to find a place you can return to regularly, so it becomes your personal retreat. Even if you're in a busy city, a park or a small green space can provide the solitude you need. Take a few minutes each day or week to reconnect with this spot, letting it become a part of your healing journey.

The key is to make this time and place sacred, wherever you find it. Nature has a way of clearing our minds, and this adaptable, outdoor practice can offer profound healing. Just find your spot, and let the journey unfold.

Sacred Scribbles *(Use these pages as a portal for decoding visions, tracking soul whispers, or just letting the ink remember what your heart already knows.)*

2

THE ESSENCE OF
SELF-EXPLORATION:
SURRENDERING TO
EXISTENTIAL GUIDEPOSTS

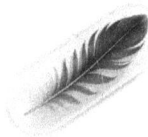

When I was four, my parents left me to spend the night at my great-aunt's studio apartment. Her bed was quartered off with bookshelves, leaving no wall of separation between us except an emotional cloud. She was a harsh woman, a piano teacher known to put a ruler under her students' wrists while they played and slap them with it if they lost the curve in their form. Her apartment had no living room furniture, only a big dining table, a piano, and a writing desk.

My bed was on the bench underneath a bay window. It provided me with a glimmer of hope to see outside, providing a respite from the gloom of the interior. Anticipating the moment my parents would pick me up the next day, I fell asleep as early as possible. When I woke up in the morning, a tiny angel, the size of a baby doll, greeted me, levitating in front of me. Witnessing quietly, I felt a surge of calm. I don't recall the angel's words, but the feeling I had told me not to fear; the angels were always with me. "Oh, wow, the angels are watching over me!" I thought as I sank back into the blanket for a minute, giddy with excitement, before I got out of bed.

I always believed in angels, but I had never met one. Angels appeared in paintings on the church ceiling, and Mom sewed my favorite cherub into a blue quilted tapestry she hung on my bedroom wall to protect me after I almost died as a baby. She told me the story of my three-year-old near-death experience many times growing up. "Your father broke the speed limit to get you to the hospital." I had epiglottitis, a life-threatening, rare condition for children in which the flap at the very back of the throat becomes swollen. The condition comes on suddenly, quickly obstructing the airways, making it hard to breathe. My face turned blue by the time we made it to the emergency room. The doctors inserted a breathing tube that saved my life.

Mom and Dad came to pick me up from my great aunt's house. When I told my mom about the angel, she smiled and listened to my story. She believed in angels, too.

I was eager to get home and tell my best friend and neighbor, Simon, about the angel. We shared the same name and our yards connected, but he had dark hair and mine was blonde. I already had my parents' approval to go to his house when my dad pulled into the driveway. I ran across the grass to knock on Simon's back door. His mom invited me to come inside. Simon was playing in the kitchen, and his parents were close by. "Guess what I saw last night?" I asked him loudly, knowing he would never guess.

"I saw an angel," I continued, out of breath from my excitement. Before Simon could respond, his parents interrupted.

"That's silly," his mom said. "You didn't see an angel. There's no such thing." She looked at his father, and they laughed.

"It was just your imagination. You were probably dreaming," his dad said.

Simon chimed in, "Yeah, that's silly." He looked at me and shrugged his shoulders.

I stood there ashamed, doing everything I could to not cry. I didn't crack. We kept playing, and all I could think about was how stupid I was for telling them what I had seen. Not a single tear fell from my eyes until I was alone in my room later that night.

The angel was a visual reality that was as real as talking to dark-haired Simon and his parents. Fifty-some odd years later, the memory has only solidified the angel's presence for me. To Simon's parents, angels didn't exist, so they thought it made sense to make sure I understood their belief was right, when it could have just as well been their illusion. They were not trying to hurt me. They saw my truth was a lie because they couldn't see it. Maybe someone told them that what they saw wasn't there when they were children.

I've grown to understand that my reaction to being told angels don't exist was to shut down. Staying quiet was a compromise that protected me from the harm and shame of proclaiming my truth.

From then on, the few times I attempted to speak my mind, I suffered the consequences, especially for meeting my needs as a husband and executive.

Meeting the angel was my first encounter with intuition. If you believe in angels, perhaps you have met your intuition. Maybe, like many kids, you were also told it was wrong.

Listening Is the Medicine

In the transition from childhood to young adulthood, our bodies are under mental and physical stress as we prepare for our independence[8]. The decision-making part of the brain is not fully developed until our mid to late twenties. When do we finally learn to listen to the physical signals our bodies send us to keep us safe?

The onset of bad information and false conditioning that we absorb in childhood and our first meetings with rejection compound in adolescence as we put social acceptance by others ahead of everything else. That small moment of being shut down by my friend Simon's parents in front of him was the beginning of the belief system that my inner guide was a liar. That moment, along with many others throughout adolescence and young adulthood, demonstrated that people would reject me if I spoke the truth. Fear of non-acceptance clouded the greatest access point to my authentic self.

Intuition meets us in a split, often fleeting second before doubt moves in, signaling what we feel is right or wrong. The art is listening to it, tuning into that moment, and prolonging your connection to your body's signals before outside information floods you. Listening to your intuition uncovers courage and the ability to decipher bad information and false conditioning from good. Pausing prevents overthinking and helps you become an active listener to your best guide. You can accept it as your God-given gift if you are spiritual. If you are not, perhaps you can see it from a scientific standpoint.

It is easy to confuse bad information and false conditioning with intuition. Bodily sensations like a racing heart, which often signal anxiety or fear, differ from the "gut feeling" that shows intuition. Creating space to stop and pay attention for a split second before responding can help you determine if you are making an empowered decision or a fearful one.

Safety makes its home in authenticity.[IP] Living out the truth of who we are sets us free, allowing us to create connections with the right people, design our professional careers to shape our strengths, and reach levels of bliss far beyond the feeling of happiness. I wasn't aware of this until after a year of struggling with the physical pain brought on by the mystery illness that began plaguing me in my late 40s. Finally, I decided to pay attention to my body's sensations after numbly going through the motions, ignoring my emotions, and forcing myself to endure the pain to avoid appearing weak. When I did, I chose a different pathway to treatment that proved successful. This was the beginning of self-exploration, and over time, I would look back at all the moments when I bypassed my authentic experience, which had appeared since I was rushed to the hospital at the age of three.

Before we know it, the obsession with outside acceptance and opinions in our adolescence transfers into a life we live with great unawareness, like the feeling of arriving somewhere by car, only to forget how we got to our destination. There's a term for this. Highway hypnosis is explained as an altered mental state in which we can drive many miles and respond to external events without being conscious.[9] This type of hypnotic state is linked to many motor vehicle accidents. The recommended antidote is to stop during a long drive, take breaks, and periodically get out of the car. Too often, we restlessly press the gas to a destination, thinking we are safe to forge on because we made it home one more time alive, without stopping. We are too distracted to notice that in acting based on false conditioning, we have forgotten what we live for.

When the Road Awakens You

When I was ten, a drunk driver hit our family car. My dad was behind the wheel. His body was squashed between the driver's side door and the middle console, breaking his hip and rupturing his bladder. My face was cut open by shards of glass that went flying from the impact. My mother had a bruised rib, and thankfully, my sister was left unscathed. The police at the scene told my dad that if the car had been hit just a few inches closer to his door, it's unlikely we would have survived.

Leading up to the accident, to save time and energy, rather than pull out of our parking spot and drive to an intersection where he could turn around, my dad took a shortcut—a 180-degree turn to get onto the main road. Even though he turned into the correct lane, the police blamed him for the illegal maneuver. The guy who hit us, who came flying down the road, had a blood alcohol level that ultimately placed the legal responsibility on him. In some way, it seemed my dad and the drunk driver were both on autopilot. If my dad had taken the time to do a legal turnaround, or the guy had decided not to get into the car after he had been drinking, none of us would have been rushed to the hospital. My dad drove carefully after that. I'm not sure if the other guy stopped drinking, but I wonder if he used the experience as an existential guidepost like Dad did.

Eight years after the car accident, I hit a patch of black ice on my motorcycle and flew headfirst into a field. The only way to see black ice is to look for points in the road that are a little darker and duller than the rest. This would require paying close attention, something most 18-year-olds on motorcycles neglect. Fortunately, I walked away with only a severely skinned leg, no broken bones, and a lot of bruises. Was I driving too fast? Could I have been paying more attention?

It's easy to think there's not enough time to pause, yet when we react too quickly, our mistakes cost us. We might find ourselves stopping to apologize, backtrack, and make up for our actions. Why are we so afraid of slowing down?

We might think we are doing the right thing when we run on tight schedules and check the boxes of accomplishment. If you are like me, you could be running away from the right kind of achievement. I worked tirelessly for money and accolades. As I ran toward the next promotion, I kept looking back for a crowd cheering me on. I didn't realize that I was seeking quick-fixes like Dad taking the shortcut or the alcohol the drunk driver drank to produce a feeling or a state of being. The lessons are hard to see in the moment but so easy to see when we pause and reflect.

THE LESSONS WE CHOOSE TO LEARN

Many of us get wrapped up in the stress of our daily lives early on. We might fear rejection and isolation, leading us to do everything possible to please others. We are being judged based on what we wear, the shape of our bodies, and how much money we have. We do what we think is necessary to fit in when what we want is to belong. Our efforts to show up in designer jeans and squeeze ourselves into an acceptable size cut off our circulation, as well as the sense of security and support we are searching for.

We can find authenticity when we speak and act in alignment with our goals, based on how we present ourselves to the world. Being authentic requires expressing our personality and spirit, no matter how pressed we feel to fit in. The deeper the roots of false conditioning that begin soon after we are born grow, the harder it is to access authenticity. Although people believe authenticity is inherently good and moral and the true self is free from outside influence, the external world becomes far more important than anything else as we grow into adolescence.

Adolescence is a time of experimentation, and the amount of rejection we experience, or lack thereof, may threaten or strengthen our intuition. The more we seek to conform, the less we act on intuition, and the further away we travel from authenticity.

Learning to differentiate between my intuition and gut reactions influenced by negative experiences and past conditioning meant I had to become attuned to bodily sensations serving as reliable indicators. Fear and anxiety make me tremble, and intuition makes me buzz. It's like the difference between drinking a jolting energy drink and a cup of green tea. It took my surrendering to the feelings to figure this out.

The epiglottitis, the drunk driver, and the motorcycle were not accidents. At three years old, I had a potential way out of the fear-based world. I had a potential way out at ten. I had a potential way out at 18, again at 46 with the onset of the mystery illness, and yet again at 50 when I was diagnosed with cancer.

After five decades of existential guideposts showing up, I began listening. I've considered how easy life would be if we were all born with a handbook laying out our soul plan with lessons we would be tasked to learn, informing us ahead of time. The whole point in living is that we get to figure this out for ourselves. We all have different timelines when we yield to our intuition and discover who we authentically are.

A **soul plan** is the spiritual belief that each soul creates a predetermined blueprint before incarnating, outlining key life experiences, challenges, and relationships to foster personal growth and evolution. Rooted in many ancient traditions like Hinduism and Buddhism, and popularized in New Age spirituality, soul plans suggest that souls choose their circumstances to learn important lessons. While free will plays a role in how these plans unfold, challenges are seen as opportunities for spiritual advancement, guided by a higher purpose and a path towards the ultimate goal: Enlightenment.

Existential guideposts are there to call us to let go. Mine eventually translated into the creation of a long and healthy life that I am consciously building for myself and others. It's not done for us easily or automatically. It's intentional and action-based. When we extract lessons from existential guideposts, it not only makes sense of our lives, but more importantly, we get the opportunity to determine how we will show up and act toward that life. The air we breathe, how we nourish our bodies, the people we spend time with, what we read, and how we speak and communicate come through as spirited acts of authenticity. We find high vibrational energy, reflective of joy, bliss, and love. We express ourselves enthusiastically. We commit to all of it because our outlook on life completely changes when we act according to our truth.

Perhaps we are all destined to surrender at a certain time that is subconsciously chosen by us. The timing aligns with the lessons we must learn to carry out our purpose. You may wonder why so many people transition from this earth, never actualizing their long, purposeful, and healthy lives. I believe it has everything to do with how open we are to exploring what I call the "illogical." This isn't about risking safety or security or being stupid or reckless. It is about letting ourselves out of the cage that keeps us from exploring all dimensions of our health, including the spiritual domain. (If you don't like the word "spiritual," I invite you to substitute the word existential.) It is about being a little "out there," because it takes thinking outside the fear-based stratosphere to find ways to heal.

Making Peace with The Past

The crescendo of my surrender happened at the brink of the return of a cancerous lump in my throat. I could no longer keep asking myself why bad things kept happening to me. Instead, I would figure out why and make peace with my past to transform tragedy into opportunity. I do not know the answer to why or how you will make peace with your tragedy, and I certainly do not know how it feels to experience the things that I have not experienced. What I know is that we are surrounded by stories of people who have been burned by fire, wrongly imprisoned, tortured, and traumatized, who created purpose and meaning out of their wounds, and used their experiences as existential guideposts rather than mere misfortune. Those are the people who motivated me to get out of bed when I was going through chemotherapy. Those are the people who kept me company during severe bouts of loneliness that mirrored some of the microtraumas that were compounded in my childhood. Upon surrendering, I went back in time to get to the root of what was plaguing me emotionally, mentally, physically, and spiritually. At the core of my dis-ease was isolation, loneliness, and an unmet need to be seen and loved unconditionally. What is at the core of what makes you uncomfortable, uneasy, fatigued, or ill?

Even though I was so young, I remember waking up from epiglottitis in the hospital in an oxygen tent surrounded by clear plastic walls. I was completely alone at that moment. Opening my eyes, I saw that my parents were not there, and there were no nurses. No one to hold me, I remember being happy to see my dad when he first appeared outside the tent. I motioned to show him where the zipper was to open the plastic. But even though he could open the tent, I had to remain in bed.

After the drunk driver hit our car, I woke up in the hospital with stitches in my head and the painful, pulsating feeling that comes with swelling. I lay there alone after another traumatic event, unable to sleep, wondering in isolation how my dad was doing and if my mother would be arriving soon.

Existential guideposts ask us to pause, look back, and make sense of it all before making our next move. They present opportunities to confront our past, repair our relationship with it, and create space to look at our lives from new and empowering vantage points. Realizing that I went through a series of events that created a deep belief that something was wrong with me and that I would be abandoned, I peeled back layers of what I learned to let go of the lies. Thinking independently brought me the courage I needed to examine my life and take responsibility for it. The examination of my life opened up a world of knowledge and possibilities.

READER REFLECTION: IDENTIFYING YOUR EXISTENTIAL GUIDEPOSTS

What life events can you look back upon and recognize as calls to move closer to authenticity, purpose, and healing?

How have your existential guideposts contributed to where you are today (both positively and negatively)?

What lessons can you extract from your existential guideposts, and how can you use them for positive change in your emotional, mental, physical, and spiritual health from this point forward?

ACTIONABLE INSIGHTS TO HEAL ACROSS FOUR DIMENSIONS OF HEALTH

Emotional

Trusting your intuition and letting go of external judgments will help you begin to reconnect with your authentic self.

Mental

Recognizing how past experiences, positive and negative, have shaped your decision-making helps neutralize how you think about them, allowing you to reframe those patterns and create a mindset of clarity and self-acceptance.

Physical

Listening to the signals and sensations your body is sending will help you figure out how to use them as a guide to making better decisions about your health and overall well-being.

Spiritual

Surrender to the lessons from your existential guideposts, allowing them to guide you toward purpose, authenticity, and spiritual growth.

SPIRITED ACT OF AUTHENTICITY: HUMAN ORACLE CARD—ACTIVATING YOUR INNER COMPASS

This ritual I have designed is inspired by the book *Dreaming with the Wheel* by Shawnodese, Sun Bear, and Wabun Wind, to help you listen to your truth.[10] This healing exercise infuses the teachings and symbolism of the medicine wheel into a practice that you can do easily from anywhere. The intention is for you to use your inner compass to tap into your intuition and use it to make decisions that help you actively create your long and healthy life. There are questions we often struggle to find the answer to. Here, I share with you a way that has helped me sit with those questions and listen to my uninterrupted and attuned inner voice, otherwise referred to as intuition.

Rooted in emotional insight and nonverbal cues, intuition enables humans to connect seemingly unrelated ideas, offering creative and innovative solutions. Some scientists now believe that the right brain activity is your natural intuition.[11] If intuition is a right-brain activity, it suggests that our intuitive abilities are closely linked to holistic thinking, creativity, and emotional intelligence. Rather than relying on linear analysis, intuition allows us to grasp the "big picture" and make decisions based on patterns or unconscious knowledge. This highlights the value of non-linear, interconnected thinking in understanding complex situations and making more emotionally attuned decisions.

The fear-based world often overrides our intuition when the left brain takes control. In that state, we can forget that we have access to truth, wisdom, and healing—simply by reconnecting with ourselves once we quiet the noise. Some call this the "Spirit" or "God" connection, or our inner knowing.

Preparation and Activation

There are several techniques to tap into our intuition, which I call our inner compass. Meditation and mindfulness are effective practices, but many struggle to stay "in the zone." I have found that simple breathing exercises can be a good way to start.

- Sit comfortably in your chair or cushion in front of your altar for a few minutes, gently breathing in and out through your nose. Just be. Have zero expectations of what is supposed to happen. Your mind will wander. Let it. Bring your awareness back to the breath, and, you guessed it, continue to just be.

- Once you become more comfortable with this, try to go for 10 minutes, then 15 minutes, then 20. Just breathe. Just be.

- At this point, you should be ready to start drawing information from the Universe, our infinite knowing, or your inner compass. You can find answers to common or uncommon life questions, such as "Should I quit my job?" "What are the next steps in restoring my relationship?" "What is the message I should be hearing today?"

Let's Get Started

- **Start by gathering information:** Before you begin your breathing technique, come up with a question your soul has been stirring up inside you. Sun Bear teaches us that the Medicine Wheel, in all its forms, has the power and the ability to connect you to infinity. Consider the infinite possible answers to your question, and allow yourself to relax to receive the answers.

  *Use the first question that comes to mind. Don't overthink it. Otherwise, your left (logical) brain will take over, and you'll miss the answer.

- **You are ready to receive the answer:** What is the first word or sentence that comes to mind? This is your answer. Again, do not overthink it or argue with it, or try to change it. There is time for contemplation and understanding. It is usually the first thought that comes to mind in a split second. Anything after that is usually the left brain trying to trick you into thinking something else.

- **Next, we move to reflection:** This is a time for quiet reflection. Take a minute to focus on the question and the answer you received. Continue to sit quietly, mentally attending to the response you were given. You may want to journal about the experience and/or write additional thoughts on paper. Is anything else stirring up? Take your time and don't rush, as this is one of the most powerful parts of the ceremony. Let your hand move freely. Don't overthink it. You might be surprised at what comes out when you don't let your left brain dictate. Once you are finished, on a separate piece of paper, write down your question and the answer(s) you have received. Once you feel this process is complete, move on to the next step.

- **It's time for "Transformation":** Take the second piece of paper with the question and answer(s) on it, fold it in half, and safely burn it over a candle, a wood-burning fireplace, or a campfire outside. Fire allows for rapid transformation. It provides the avenue to let go of old stories and trauma, to transform, renew, and rebirth. Calmly place your attention on the fire, and ask *Spirit* to help you let go and allow the "how-to" to show up, releasing and transforming the original question (trauma or life situation).

  Please be careful: Have some copper or metal tongs at hand to hold the paper over the flame, and a fireproof bowl or pan ready to catch the burning paper once it lights. By releasing these old patterns and beliefs into the fire, you heal at the depth of the soul without having to experience them at the literal and physical levels.

- **Finally, you are ready for purification:** This is a time to purify your intentions, and to invite the spirit guidance to be with you as you go about your day or start to wind down for the night. The best form of purification is water. I love stepping barefoot into the stream behind my house and washing my hands and face. Do the same if you can access a stream or lake, or opt for a salt bath at home by dissolving Epsom salt, Himalayan salt, or sea salt in the bath water. As an alternative, you can simply splash your face with refreshing cold water.

Sacred Scribbles *(Use these pages as a portal for decoding visions, tracking soul whispers, or just letting the ink remember what your heart already knows.)*

3

FINDING FORGIVENESS:
EXTENDING GRACE TO
OUR INNER AND OUTER
ADVERSARIES

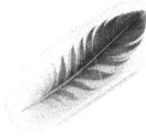

B elonging can only happen in a State of Authenticity. In adolescence, trying to fit in only strengthens the false conditioning. It's a time when many of us move further from our truth, as we crave acceptance from our peers. As children or adults, we are unique and distinct when genuine. Each one of us stands alone in our eccentricities. Rather than embracing what makes us stand out from others, we try to make ourselves more appealing to them, in hopes of making friends or joining social groups. When we apply but don't get approved for membership, we further our quest to conform to what we see others saying and doing.

Studies have shown that social rejection activates the same areas of the brain as physical pain.[12] This indicates that rejection hurts more than we might currently comprehend.

Adolescent insecurities and low self-esteem can make us feel on edge, anxious, and maybe even destructive of ourselves or others as we develop into adulthood. There are micro moments of rejection, like my Grandma Ingrid leaving me alone in her living room, or Simon's parents laughing at me, telling me the angel wasn't real. There are macro moments of rejection that carve through our psyche, entering through the little scratches on the surface and finding a home in the chasms of our bodies. If we decide to use rejection as a catalyst for change, or even better, a transformation, then we must come face-to-face with our adversaries, including ourselves. Healthy confrontation of self means we move conflict, injustice, shame, remorse, and guilt out of our system to make space for forgiveness and grace. This, I believe, indicates we are practicing self-love, opening the doors of our hearts up to belonging, acceptance, and appreciation.

The Cost of Fitting In

In rural Switzerland, the buses didn't come for the kids who lived a short distance from the school. Starting in kindergarten, we began walking to school without our parents chaperoning us. On the surface, it felt safe to walk unaccompanied by an adult because we lived in a place without crime, a place where the community was seemingly well-adjusted, with no outward present dangers. Most days, it was Fritz, a bigger kid a year older than me, a small five-year-old girl named Beatrix, and me who walked together. Early in the year, on our way to school, Fritz began shoving Beatrix into a field, knocking her down. This happened daily, with him laughing at her before trudging onward without looking back. I tried to ignore Fritz, hoping that by not paying attention to his behavior, he would stop. Unfortunately for Beatrix, that didn't happen. Before long, he invited me to participate. Wanting to avoid the two of us, Beatrix's mission began early to keep ahead of us. She walked as fast as her little legs could take her, but that didn't help. Her short legs simply weren't as long as ours, which meant we could easily catch up to her. Fritz watched and goaded me on as I shoved her. He stood behind me as if to say he had my back. I had convinced my inner self that I was powerful. This perception was the only way I believed I could remain safe from being beaten by Fritz. I told myself he wouldn't harm me as long as I continued to harm Beatrix.

For a few weeks, this became a game I played. Fritz and I would tease and shove Beatrix into the field before running through the school's doors and taking our seats unscathed. The walks continued to look the same until one day, Beatrix's mom joined her. As I approached, her mom noticed me, stopped, then sternly motioned for me to come closer. I knew enough to listen to adults and obliged.

"You look at this," I recall her mother saying sternly as she lifted Beatrix's pant leg to expose her scraped leg with a large, black, and blue bruise. What must she have felt at that moment, looking at the boy who left marks on her sweet little girl?

Horrified, I realized that I had done something very wrong. Immediately, I felt sick and remorseful.

"You did this!" Her stare darted directly into mine.

I didn't look away from her. I cannot remember what more was said, and I won't attempt to make it up. I knew at that moment that I regretted hurting Beatrix. I felt shame for playing along, and I resolved never to hurt or shove her again. At some point, I believe her mother put enough fear into Fritz that he, too, stopped bullying Beatrix because it all came to an end. Maybe Fritz felt ashamed, just like I did. I didn't see him much after that, but I've wondered what his home life was like and whether someone was hurting him.

Unfortunately, I cannot tell the story you might be hoping to hear, and one that I wish I could tell. The one where I stood up to Fritz and shoved him into the field, took Beatrix by the hand, and became a hero. No, I was a coward. I participated. I let fear convince me that it was the only way; the bullying had to continue. Her mother never contacted my parents, so they never served any consequences. It seemed as though I had no repercussions, so I could conveniently hide the fact that, for a short amount of time, I was a bully. Little did they know I would be plagued by my own actions, lack of consequences, and unanswered questions. If they knew what I did to Beatrix, would I still be loved? What will people think of me? Why did I allow fear to control me? Am I like Fritz?

Walking to and from school remained peaceful until two years later. There were several boys I called my friends. I encountered both of them at the end of the school day along the route back to my house. Like me, Christian and Samuel were in the second grade. I was excited that the cast of schoolmates I walked with every day had changed. But what originally looked like an opportunity for me to form friendships quickly became a dysfunctional triangle of torture that I falsely identified as friendship. Walking past Christian's house, Samuel would already be there. The two of them would run out and invite me to come over. On the safe days, we would play and laugh, and I would make it home unscathed. More often, during the time I spent at Christian's, I would be wrestled in a headlock, tormented, and beaten up. Because I wanted their friendship so badly, I kept accepting the invitation to come over, holding out hope for the day the bullying would stop.

I tried to devise a secret plan to fight back by reading my dad's books on karate and Jiu-Jitsu, thinking I needed to battle for respect. The desire to fight back unleashed a hidden, primal aggression in me, but I wasn't a martial artist or a street fighter. I was a little kid who wanted to be friends with the wrong people. Eventually, I put the books down, and Christian and Samuel turned their attention to bullying others. I turned mine into girls.

My first love was a Greek girl named Alexia. We were both eight, but she looked much older. Towering over me, I fell in love with her grandiosity. Every day, I would escort her to pick up her brother from his after-school program, then walk them both home. But she was walking me, as I fawned over her the whole way. It was clear we had a crush on one another, but when she asked me to kiss her, I knew exactly where I stood, tall enough to reach her chin. She took off the winter ski mask I was wearing and exposed my red cheeks. Shaking from my nerves and the cold, I lifted my heels as high as possible to meet her halfway. She bent down and tenderly placed her lips on my cheek. That was my first kiss from a girl who wasn't my mom or sister. After that, we continued to school and made plans to meet at the end-of-year dance coming up.

Arriving at the dance, I settled in but didn't see Alexia anywhere. The music had started, so I figured she would be waiting for me somewhere nearby. Scanning around the perimeter of the gymnasium, I couldn't find her anywhere. Shifting my gaze to the dance floor, there she was, swaying back and forth with her hands around the neck of my so-called friend Noah. Upset, I fled, crying, running home to my mom. When I made it through the front door, I was hyperventilating, tears streaming down my face. Trying to explain what happened amidst my rapid breaths, I shared that Alexia had broken up with me. As silly as it sounds now, even though I find the sweetness and the humor looking back on this experience, I located the root of another layer of isolation that began compounding the illusion that I wasn't worthy of love, and the little scratches were deepening the wounds. In the coming decades, I was rejected by women, wondering if I would ever find my wife.

Forty-eight years after terrorizing Beatrix, I ran into her at a class reunion in our hometown. "Simon, this is my little sister Beatrix." It turned out that a woman I had been introduced to before the reunion, who was a few years older than me, was Beatrix's older sister. When she reintroduced us, not knowing that we had already met, Beatrix and I looked at one another, and we knew that neither of us had forgotten what had happened. As an adult, I always wondered if she carried those bruises forward into the rest of her life. In front of our adult friends, I immediately began acknowledging what happened and apologizing.

"Oh, you were that kid?!" her sister asked, shocked. The others stood there, looking at me with distaste. I didn't blame them. I blamed myself, but the disapproving looks transported me back into the body of my six-year-old self, the boy following the leader in hopes of being seen, the boy who would do anything to feel loved and accepted, even if that meant pushing an innocent little girl. I carried on with my apology, blocking out the onlookers to focus on the exchange between Beatrix and me.

There was no more hiding. As uncomfortable as it was to reveal at fifty that I was one of her bullies, I fell in love with her in our gentle exchange. This is a love story, but not the one you might anticipate.

No More Secrets

The act of admitting I was the former bully of Beatrix was an act of self-love—no more hiding. My intuition told me to be open with her when expressing my apologies. Beatrix and I engaged in conversation. She explained that she did not think much about our pushing and shoving her before seeing me. Her life was well-adjusted. Sharing with me that she is a nurse, I understood that the little girl who got hurt was now working to mend the pain of others.

"Forgive yourself, Simon. I've forgiven you." I was relieved that she wasn't suffering because of my actions and amazed by the compassion she had toward me. Forgiveness is a fortunate gift that we are not always granted by others. Forgiveness is an act we must do with and for ourselves, whether others participate; yet when they do, it provides evidence that there are people who can see right through to the core of who we are.

Fessing up to being the bully, I reached a point where there were no more secrets in my life. Vocalizing my truth and even writing it down here to share with you, I admit that I still hear a whisper of fear in my ear, telling me that maybe you will stop reading, that a friend will shun me, or that a client won't work with me if I admit to wrongdoing in my past. Then I ask myself, "What does life look like when there are no more secrets? When everything is on the table?" Liberating. Free. Unobstructed. Safe.

There is nothing you can't ask me or that I can't talk about because those whispers of fear are so small compared to the love that comes through after I empty my pockets of shame. To think we will not be loved if we own up to our mistakes is an illusion. Moments like the one I had with Beatrix at our reunion have proven that in authenticity, love boomerangs back to us in the most surprising ways. When we feel like no one will love us if we show the less appealing parts of ourselves, someone shows up to prove us wrong.

I decided I could have faith that if I were course-correcting, listening to the existential guideposts, and working to become congruent in every area of my life, that alignment would free me from false conditioning and bad information. Learning and unlearning were the roots of my emotional, intellectual, physical, and spiritual healing.

At the end of the day, we have to answer to ourselves. It's you and only you who know the truth of your heart. No one can hurt you more than you can hurt yourself. Relentless rumination and condemnation of oneself due to guilt, shame, and remorse will not set anyone free. Gossip culture may challenge you. Righteous people might feel threatened by you. Rest assured, they have to answer to themselves at the end of the day, too.

Seeing Beatrix later in life was unplanned, but it was perfect timing. We are all looking for unconditional love, which comes to us in the most surprising moments. I like to believe that it is delivered by others after we have shown it to ourselves, so we are open to receiving it.

All the walking back and forth from school to home was filled with enemies and antagonists, including myself, high on false conditioning and bad information. We do a version of this walk every single day, going in and out of trigger moments in a world that scares us back into place, before we finally turn and face the lady we cut off in traffic, the boss who demoted us, or, more importantly, the little child within us that is waiting for us to release all of it from our system, so we can come out and play. Stay committed; the world will look at you with eyes of grace and unconditional love.

READER REFLECTION: IDENTIFYING YOUR MICRO AND MACRO TRAUMAS

Looking back on your childhood, what painful moments have you left unprocessed because they felt insignificant?

Over the course of your childhood, what, if any, bigger events or secrets have you held inside or left unprocessed because they felt too big to confront?

If you were to visualize yourself healed from the micro and macro traumas in your life, what would become possible for you? How would life look, smell, taste, sound, and feel different?

ACTIONABLE INSIGHTS TO HEAL ACROSS FOUR DIMENSIONS OF HEALTH

Emotional

Facing past mistakes and extending forgiveness to yourself and others allows you to release guilt and experience emotional freedom.

Mental

Confronting the harmful beliefs you've internalized from micro and macro traumas helps reframe them in a way that fosters self-acceptance and mental clarity.

Physical

By acknowledging how holding onto shame or remorse affects your body and practicing forgiveness, you can free yourself from physical tension and distress.

Spiritual

Embracing authenticity by admitting your past wrongdoings and extending grace to yourself opens you up to love and spiritual growth.

SPIRITED ACT OF AUTHENTICITY: CRADLED AND HELD—HEALING MICRO TRAUMAS ASSOCIATED WITH LONELINESS

What if, as children, no matter what we did, love was at the forefront?

What if we treat ourselves that way as adults?

If a child smashes a window, rather than being yelled at for doing something wrong, what if we are met with love and a parent who works with us to right the wrong?

What if the parent places her arm around the child and says, "Let's go find the owner of that window and confess?"

In love, there are still consequences when we don't do the right thing. There has to be because love cares enough to stop and pay attention to the heart of the issue, and it takes time to understand.

Here, I invite you to re-parent your inner child by cradling and holding your little self. The focus is on loneliness and associated feelings. Experiment with this exercise, using other feelings based on your realizations as you look back. Use your stories to grow and shift how you interact with the world around you.

Cradled and Held is an exercise in exploring the depths of your inner child to harness the power of your past experiences for healing and growth. This lesson is designed for you to seek peace with your traumatic childhood and utilize those experiences as stepping stones toward a more fulfilling present and future.

Acknowledge the Wounds: Begin by acknowledging the wounds of your inner child. Reflect on the micro and macro experiences that shaped you, both positive and negative. Allow yourself to feel the emotions associated with those memories without judgment or suppression. Understand that these wounds are a part of your story, but do not define your worth or potential.

Embrace Compassion: Extend compassion to your inner child. Visualize yourself cradling your younger self in a warm, nurturing embrace. Offer words of comfort and reassurance, acknowledging the pain while affirming your strength and resilience. Practice self-compassion by treating yourself with kindness and understanding.

Reclaim Your Power: Identify how past experiences have shaped your beliefs, behaviors, and self-perception. Challenge any limiting beliefs or negative patterns that may have stemmed from childhood trauma. Take back control of your narrative by reframing your story with empowering perspectives. You are not defined by what happened to you; you are defined by how you choose to respond and grow.

Integrate and Transform: Integrate the lessons learned from your inner child into your daily life. Apply newfound insights and self-awareness to positively change your relationships, career, and overall well-being. Embrace the transformative power of healing, knowing that each step forward brings you closer to wholeness and authenticity.

As you complete the Cradled and Held lesson, remember that healing is a lifelong journey filled with ups and downs. Be gentle with yourself and celebrate your progress along the way. By embracing your inner child and honoring your past experiences, you pave the way for a brighter, more resilient future. You are worthy of love, health, and joy.

Sacred Scribbles *(Use these pages as a portal for decoding visions, tracking soul whispers, or just letting the ink remember what your heart already knows.)*

PART 2. LOVE

CALIBRATING YOUR NAVIGATION SYSTEM

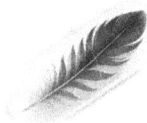

Love is something you and I must have. We must have it because our spirit feeds upon it. We must have it because without it, we become weak and faint. Without love, our self-esteem weakens. Without it, our courage fails. Without love, we can no longer look out confidently at the world.

—Chief Dan George (Tsleil-Waututh Nation)

During my time of illness, I had the profound privilege of learning from the paqos, specifically from Don Juan, a Q'ero shaman. He often performed ceremonies accompanied by the soothing sounds of his flute or rattle. His music carried a deep, calming energy, pulling me into a trance-like state where I was enveloped in stillness and peace. As I watched him work, I realized that his mere presence—his quiet, unassuming nature—was a kind of healing in itself. It was in that space of pure contentment that I found myself reflecting on what it truly means to be in alignment with our highest self and the world around us.

This experience of pure presence, of love in action, was a catalyst in my journey to becoming a Neo-shaman, a messenger for the Q'ero. Neo-shamanism, while drawing from traditional practices, adapts these ancient teachings for our modern lives. I was determined to find practical applications that could help me and others find peace in a chaotic and disconnected world. There were many surprising realizations along the way.

One such lesson came during a healing ceremony, where Don Juan spat water in my face. At first, I misunderstood. I was taken aback and, admittedly, somewhat offended. It felt rude, disrespectful even—certainly not the kind of act one associates with a blessing. Little did I know, this wasn't just any water—it was Agua de Florida, a sacred water used in Indigenous rituals for cleansing, blessing, and protection. When it hit my skin, I felt the shock of it—the discomfort of having something spat on me. Initially, I questioned the meaning behind it, and my Western conditioning led me to think it was an insult.

As I remained still and present, I realized that the discomfort itself was part of the lesson. I wasn't meant to retreat or react in anger. I was invited to stay with the discomfort, to be present with the feelings that arose, and in doing so, I opened myself to a deeper understanding of healing and love.

I learned a powerful lesson about unconditional love. True love does not shy away from discomfort. True love does not avoid the difficult moments or the messy, uncomfortable parts of ourselves and others. Instead, it invites us to stay, to hold space, and to allow for transformation. This is the essence of unconditional love—not just loving ourselves when we are perfect or comfortable, but embracing all parts of ourselves, especially the parts that may feel vulnerable or unworthy.

As you read these pages, I invite you to reflect on what it might have felt like to have water spat on your face in the way I experienced with Agua de Florida. Sometimes, love is not the soft, easy feeling we often expect.

Unconditional embraces imperfections. Through the teachings of the paqos and my own experiences, I have come to understand that healing, at its core, is the process of learning to love ourselves unconditionally, even in our most vulnerable moments. This kind of love opens the door for us to give and receive love freely, without expectations, without judgment, and without fear.

Just as Agua de Florida is used to cleanse and bless, consider how your own challenges with others might be sacred moments for healing. The practice of unconditional love, both for ourselves and for others, may be exactly what you need to welcome the transformation that awaits.

STORY FROM THE HEALING TABLE: RELEASING UNHEALTHY ATTACHMENTS

We fear dying alone, yet we tend to live our lives in pursuit of lust, attachment, and validation, which leaves us lacking genuine connection. True love is not dependent on giving and receiving based on expectations. Offering love only if granted something in return keeps us stuck in a low-vibrational reactionary system, an endless loop of feeling let down.

Love is a response, not a reaction.[IP] A reaction is immediate, driven by the unconscious mind's beliefs and biases. It happens without conscious thought, focusing on survival and defense, often leading to regret. In contrast, a response is more deliberate, drawing from the conscious and unconscious mind. It considers long-term effects and the well-being of others, aligning with core values. While reactions and responses may appear similar, their underlying motivations and outcomes differ significantly. A response tends to be more thoughtful, compassionate, and measured, aiming for a balanced and beneficial impact.

When Lisa, a young woman in her twenties, came to my healing table, she explained to me that she was experiencing a lack of focus, mental clarity, and enthusiasm for life. The lethargy, she told me, had made it difficult for her to get out of bed most mornings. Aware enough to know that this was not her normal way of being, she was unable to come up with an explanation as to why this was happening to her. As I asked her a series of questions, I discovered that she had recently parted ways with her former boyfriend. The most reasonable explanation for why she was having difficulty was that she was lovesick.

Lovesickness is not a diagnosed condition but a biological reaction to loss.[13] At some point in our lives, all of us have come down with this curable condition that often includes tormenting, ruminating thoughts as we recount the events leading up to a breakup, a lack of motivation, insomnia, and isolation. The symptoms vary from person to person, depending on the unique dynamics of the relationship, but the feelings of despair and longing are universal. We might skip meals or indulge in comfort food because our gut—our emotional core—is unwell, triggering our minds to deny or fill the void.

More than likely, you have heard a story about a widow or widower passing away soon after their spouse. While these stories seem to tug at our hearts as we think of one person being unable to go on without the other because they were deeply in love, there might be more to it. One particularly interesting study by a group of behavioral medical professionals found that the health of partners is considerably interconnected.[14] It also found that the couples' health risks, when combined, can be greater than if they were single. The point is that, if these studies are correct, love can make us so sick that our lives might even be threatened. My counterpoint is that the cure is to uncondition ourselves from the bad information and false ideas we have adopted about love to rid ourselves of the affliction.

Lisa was grieving, attached to the energetic cord, or spiritual tether, of the relationship with her ex. Through years of seeing similar "conditions" in my practice, I knew that having an energetic cord attached to her was one of the symptoms ailing her, but there was more dragging her down than her recent breakup.

The term **energetic cord** does not have a singular, traceable origin but emerges from various spiritual and metaphysical traditions, blending concepts from Eastern philosophies like the subtle body and prana (life force) with New Age and Neo-Shamanic practices. These traditions focus on the idea of unseen energy exchanges between individuals or entities, which can impact emotional, spiritual, and physical well-being. Neo-Shamanism, in particular, popularized the concept of cord-cutting as a way to sever harmful energetic connections, adapting ideas from ancient shamanic healing practices. I highly recommend one of my favorite books on this topic, *Energy Strands* by author Denise Lynn, if you would like to take your learning and love to the next level.15

Before I began my work with Lisa, my friend and teacher, Peter Bonaker, informed me of a recently discovered phenomenon most likely to blame for the additional lack of focus and lethargy that Lisa complained about. Some of Peter's former academic colleagues laughed at him when he first discovered this, a year before he shared it with me. He ended up writing a book about the "Sacred Shield," in which he describes a "dark, malevolent, energetic form that seems to be attaching itself to people between the physical and the spiritual auric field."[16] What sounds a bit like science fiction is very real to me. I've seen time and time again that when someone is spiritually attacked by this energetic form, depression, anxiety, panic attacks, lack of direction, and physical ailments, including cold shivers, are typical symptoms. Once this energetic connection is removed and someone is back in their own body without foreign interference, the panic attacks and mental challenges stop.

Have you ever felt an uncomfortable feeling in another person's presence that you can't explain? How about a feeling of intense excitement or connection? What you're feeling is their invisible auric field touching yours. When the vibration of the person doesn't match yours, then it's like two magnets with the same polarity pushing each other away. When it does, it's like two batteries touching opposite poles that turn on a flashlight.

An **auric field** is the subtle energy surrounding the body, reflecting one's emotional, mental, physical, and spiritual state, with layers vibrating at different frequencies. In Shamanism, this field is seen as a dynamic energy matrix that can absorb or project energy, and its balance is essential for overall well-being. To cleanse the auric field, neo-shamans use rituals like smudging with sage or other sacred herbs, sound healing through drums or tuning forks, and energy extractions to remove blockages and restore harmony in the energy body.

On the healing table, Lisa described the physical sensations in her body as I performed what I can only describe as spiritual heart surgery on her. Together, we identified unhealthy emotional attachments that went as far back as five years old that were lodged in her body and needed to be removed. The source of her pain was not as obvious as her recent breakup. In my experience, there are always layers below the surface that need to be healed. Lisa's case was no different.

When it comes to lovesickness, circling back in time to heal, we can discover that it is not only directly related to the relationship we are mourning today. It is an interconnected dis-ease. The way we observe love play out as small children, and the micro and macro traumas of our past, are behind the symptoms. A current event is the trigger, not the root cause. Lisa was holding on to her ex because she had unconsciously associated that relationship with others she hadn't fully processed. We worked through this and removed the bonds that were breaking her heart.

The immediate positive effect of being back in her own body was that she felt "like herself again." She was able to get up in the morning and go about her daily routine with ease. In time, she knew when she was free of this energetic form and when it returned.

In my professional experience, people who are not in congruence with their life's purpose or those on the verge of doing something remarkable for the common good seem to be most affected by this energy. I am often asked where this energy is coming from and who or what is behind it. I leave the answer up to interpretation. The nuances arise in the conversations between me and my clients. To me, it's all about restoring emotional and mental well-being, to allow the physical body to heal and the nervous system to calm down. Unhealthy attachments of all types drain us of our ability to love.

To be loved, we must accept that we need not ask for anything in return, and believe that if we come from a place of authenticity, love will return to us in the most surprising ways. Love doesn't ask us to change who we are. It invites us to evolve into better versions of ourselves. To stop smoking or start eating more vegetables is a reasonable request that might be incredibly difficult to implement, but changing a habit does not conflict with authenticity. Making healthier choices might even move us closer to our true identity.

Through asking questions, knowledge, and compassion, we see ourselves and others through sickness and health without asking them to be someone they are not. We live the full scope of our emotions, get unstuck, and trust that the fuel for dis-ease in our relationship with ourselves and others has to be unconditional to flourish. Conditional love, which is not love at all, is based on expectations that create transactional experiences: "I'll give you this if you give me that." Unconditional love, on the other hand, craves knowledge, looks you in the eye, and encourages everyone to grow. How do we love and allow love to come to us unconditionally?

If you think back on any tough situation, what did you need? It's always about love. It's never about the money, the status, or what people think of you. It's an urgency to know, "Will I still be loved?" When we focus on getting to the root of what is making us ill and out of congruence in our lives, there's a ton of truth given to us. Part of that is trusting that we will be loved unconditionally, on a higher level than we ever knew possible.

The last time I worked with Lisa, she told me that it felt like a switch had flipped back on when she walked out of the room. She is thinking and seeing clearly again. Energy is medicine, and the heart will launch into the stratosphere if we dance in orbit with the light.

4

UNCONDITIONING YOUR HEART: ACTIVATING LIMITLESS RELATIONSHIPS

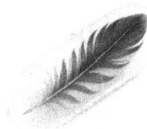

One of the most misinterpreted bible verses might be Mark 12:31: "Thou shalt love thy neighbor as thy-self." Growing up in the Lutheran church, I often heard this second biblical commandment. I interpreted it to mean that we must love others more than and before we love ourselves. This translation falls short of the emphasis this passage places on self-love. Certainly, Jesus would not want us to love ourselves only a little. That would mean we could only love others a little. Is it safe to say that self-love is the essence of the second commandment? I think so.

In our quest to find belonging and acceptance from others, we often neglect to figure out what it looks like to become more intimate with ourselves. When the world doesn't show up for us the way we wish it would, we might wonder what we lack and begin looking in the wrong places. We seek what we believe to be love by trying to make more money, filling our houses with material things, and taking on the responsibility for the happiness of everyone around us. We often aim to please those in our lives, including those not close to us, and dismiss our enjoyment of pleasure as shameful or self-centered.

The health of our hearts becomes contingent on the swinging pendulum of harsh criticism or glowing accolades received from the world around us. When we wipe ourselves clean of the vandalization of our hearts, the pure art of who we are comes to the surface. If we don't, we risk never grasping what it feels like to love from a place of authenticity.

My wife and I asked for all the wrong things from one another—at least, that was my experience. We both wanted the other to be an entirely different person from the one we married. We met at a Bon Jovi concert. She was a singer in a band, and I was a sound engineer. Our love of music brought us together before the arrival of our two children. After the kids were born, we left our careers in the arts to secure financially stable jobs, ensuring our children's safety. She became a nurse, and I entered the corporate world. Our schedules had little overlap. We thought managing childcare in shifts would be beneficial for raising the kids. With very little time we could spend together as a couple, I now understand that this was harmful to our union. Without intending to do so, we began leading separate lives.

When we did come together, our criticisms of one another replaced the long talks over dinner we once had. We were drowning in mundane nagging that kept us from enjoying the small, everyday pleasures of life. Even cooking our favorite dish together, a point of pleasure and connection in our relationship, became problematic. Our expectations of marriage, fueled by bad information and false conditioning, made us a resentful pair. She suddenly began expressing that she "hated" how I cut the green onions the recipe called for. I hated that she hated the way I cut the green onions. An endless cycle ensued. I felt homesick for the good times when we would laugh over that same meal. What happened to us?

While I continued to explore my musical side by playing the drums with the band at the church we attended, my drum set at home was coated with dust. In the passionless pursuit of possessions that we thought would bring us happiness, the music we made as individuals that had brought us together died. For a time, I went through the motions of going to work – eat – sleep – repeat, accepting that my primary role at home was to provide financial security.

I became "too busy" to notice that my tendencies to please others and provide for my family financially were making me sick. When the possibility of death kept showing up through physical illness, I knew I had to do something different if I was to maintain the hope of living a long and healthy life. Little did I know that doing something different would lead to changing almost everything.

Thinking that I was wronged by my wife was a narrative I had to change. I looked for her to repair what felt broken in me, when what I needed was self-reflection on the part I played in our unhappy marriage. Maybe she felt the pressure of what I was asking from her, just as I felt like her expectations of me to be a provider had placed a lot of pressure on me. I agreed to play the role, but underneath the surface, I blamed her for it. I'm sure she felt she had to play a role, too. It was my responsibility to form my identity as a father and husband. I knew I needed to see myself as a whole human again. I had let the logic of the outside world direct my work, my relationships, and my health. It was time to become the lead expert on my health and life.

The Roots of Love

The "love hormone," oxytocin, which bonds humans by activating trust, finding psychological stability, and relaxation, is not only produced in our social interactions. It is also created through acts of self-love and compassion. Why have we become increasingly obsessed with being attractive to others more than being satisfied with what we see in the mirror? Love hormones surge when we are shown a picture of someone we are attracted to, yet when we look at a picture of ourselves, it's often easier to point to our flaws than what makes us beautiful.

Misguided beliefs about what love looks like and how to show up and express love hurt our connections.

"She will love me if I buy the house she wants."

"I will be a good father if my children excel in school."

"My boss will promote me if I work overtime every weekend."

The conditional "ifs" we place on life clog our energetic sinks by thinking we need to do or achieve something to be admired and embraced. Looking back on my childhood, I remember times when I felt loved and cared for.

Growing up in Switzerland as a young boy, Sunday mornings were sacred for my family. Mom, Dad, my brother, the twins, and I would gather around the table to eat a late breakfast. Classical music was playing. I listened as they spoke of the teachings of Elisabeth Kübler-Ross on the psychology of death and dying, as well as philosophies that seemed far too complex for a six-year-old to understand. Little did I know that the intellectual conversations between my parents and eldest siblings would subconsciously influence my future. My mother filled the table with homemade bread, farm-fresh jams, honey, cheese, and yogurt, planting seeds for my love of cooking with whole, organic foods. Those feel-good mornings gave me a sense of unity, safety, and security. This provided me with a foundation of love in the days when I was bullied and rejected by the kids at school. I had a place where I belonged on those Sunday mornings, even after staying at my great-aunt's house or with Grandma Ingrid.

I believe that if a person has suffered a great amount of distress due to the low-vibrational energy generated by extreme abuse and trauma, there is always a high-vibrational energy buried under the rubble. Although it can be difficult to uncover the people, places, and moments that have brought us joy, doing so allows us to use those memories as proof that we can create more positive experiences. Instead of longing for old times, we create a bigger future.

As I became an independent adult, my relationship with my parents changed. The kind of person I was becoming seemed to matter less and less to them. What I did for a living mattered more. My belief in a world I could only see through their eyes, which began developing in childhood, strengthened. They taught me not to question their vision of my future, so I didn't.

With the transition into adulthood, the inquisitiveness, understanding, and compassion I felt in early childhood began to be replaced by misunderstandings and duty. To be loved and accepted, I began forming my life around what I thought would please others, staying quiet to make my presence easier for them, and fulfilling obligations as a husband, father, and corporate executive.

To be worthy of love and attention, I understood that my business card should be embossed with words indicating that I am the "Chief" of something or, at a minimum, "President." I opted for a career that proved my success instead of one that held personal significance. I was convinced that the world would compensate me with wealth and a partner who would love me unconditionally if I did what I was told I should do. My actions and reactions were reflections of the fear-based world I had over-consumed.

Rising Above the Noise

Low-vibrational energy emerges from our past wounds and unhealed experiences, manifesting as reactions like Shame ("I am fundamentally flawed"), Guilt ("I've done something unforgivable"), and Fear ("Something terrible will happen"). These reactions are based on survival mechanisms that once protected us but now keep us trapped in cycles of self-protection and limitation. When we remain in these states, whether through chronic worry, resentment, or self-criticism, we operate from a place of scarcity and defensiveness, unable to access our full potential.

High-vibrational energy begins with courage, i.e., the willingness to face our fears and take aligned action despite them. This shifts us into neutrality, where we can observe without judgment, then into acceptance of what is. From this foundation, we naturally move toward states of love, joy, and profound peace. High-vibrational responses like Reason ("I understand why this happened"), Peace ("I appreciate what this taught me"), and Love ("I am supported") are rooted in wisdom and clarity. Free from the distortions of past trauma and false beliefs, they create space for hope, meaning, and genuine transformation.[17]

Both low and high vibe energies display how communication with ourselves, others, and even inanimate objects like food, beverages, and the plants in our house can transform our health and well-being. We can have a positively charged energetic exchange (response system) with everybody and everything we can see and not see. If only one person acts from a place of compassion, the exchange cannot transcend the fear-based world until everyone participates in vibrating higher.

Unconditional love is based on moving through both high- and low-vibrational emotions. When facing struggle, having difficult conversations, or navigating low-vibrational emotions like anger, grief, or shame, it fosters a resilient kind of love that trusts we can get through the tough stuff. From there, we can fall forward, arms open wide, and be intimate with others. The best place to start raising our vibe is within, by letting go of the scarcity rooted in the belief that being true to ourselves will lead to rejection or disappointment.

We can create new muscle memories through internal cooperation that overrides the infighting and conflict we feel when we are stuck in a loop of denial, destruction, and obstruction. We must cultivate this within ourselves to be better at creating it in every aspect of our lives. Giving and receiving as a way of responsiveness helps us become more confident in listening, trusting our intuition, and paying attention to the existential guideposts as they arise.

The Illogical Path

The day I took my health into my hands, I began cultivating a new relationship with responsiveness that paved the way to opening myself up to the true love I was missing. Today, I know that this is work that takes continuous and mindful monitoring to keep my energy clean. Confronting the fear-based world is not a destination. It is a process that brings to light new layers of self that can be surprising and worthy of attention.

The deconditioning of the organ that pumps blood into our veins opens our physical, emotional, mental, and spiritual well-being, making space to renew vows of self-love. The fact is, there is only one marriage that's guaranteed to last a lifetime— the one with our own authentic self. We can choose to fight or flourish in it. If we choose to quarrel, the lies we tell ourselves take up space in our bodies, creating low-vibrational response systems that spin out of control, making us sick and tired.

The sudden onset of my autoimmune disease began on a church mission trip to the Dominican Republic that I took with my son. Out of nowhere, extreme pain suddenly struck my right shoulder, making it difficult to make even the most minor moves, like getting in and out of vehicles. Returning home, I started a new job in leisure travel. There was no relaxation in my life. The pain spread and intensified, prompting me to seek medical attention.

The doctors, having trouble diagnosing me, put me on the steroid prednisone, which muted the pain temporarily, but caused excessive weight gain and heart palpitations. The top physicians in the world continued to struggle to find out what was wreaking havoc on my body, ruling out various conditions before giving me the bullshit diagnosis of an autoimmune disease called seronegative inflammatory arthritis. It was simply a way to say, "Your body is inflamed," which I already knew. My fingers were so swollen that my hand appeared to be closed shut. The Western medical community could not figure out the root cause of what was ailing me. Going in and out of doctor visits was like dumping water on an oil fire. A low vibe had taken over my health and every aspect of my life.

Out of options, the doctor's final attempt to help me was by prescribing me a malaria drug. He recommended that, before I take it, I see an ophthalmologist because the side effects were known to lead to blindness. "Okay, doc, my eyes are the only thing working right now, so why would I mess with that?" I asked him. He never answered the question. At that point, the only thing I had was my vision.

A couple of days after that appointment with the doctor, I boarded a plane from New York to Phoenix for a work trip. I was still contemplating whether I should consider the medication because I knew I was running out of options. Sitting down in my seat, I noticed the guy next to me. He wore a hat that read "McIntosh," which immediately caught my attention. No, this had nothing to do with computers. Having spent time working as a sound engineer in the years before the kids were born, I was a fan of McIntosh Amplifiers. I rarely initiate a conversation with someone on an airplane, but I couldn't help myself. The musician in me was curious about what he did for a living. In mere seconds, we were immersed in a personal conversation. I told him about what I was going through.

"I was recently diagnosed with seronegative inflammatory arthritis." He looked at me in disbelief. "That was my wife's diagnosis," he said. "She was prescribed a type of malaria medication and, after taking it, developed Lupus. She passed away five years later. "They just prescribed me malaria medication," I told him. We confirmed it was the same medication. This was a chance encounter that gave me everything I needed to know to make my decision. If I hadn't been sitting next to him, I probably would have filled the prescription. I had gone as far as I could within what I now call the "logical spaces" to heal.

My frustration stemmed from being misdiagnosed—and from the Western medical system's inability to provide answers. I realized that there are so many people like me. When you live with chronic illnesses and unexplained symptoms, you feel dismissed—not just by the medical system, but also by friends and family. They make comments like, *"Hey, you look fine. What's wrong with you? You don't look sick."* I understand that it's hard for people to change what they've been taught about what a sick person looks like, but it doesn't make it any easier.

Meeting this man on the plane, I felt very strongly that I had to stop putting band-aids on the symptoms and do the work to get to the root of what was plaguing me. The warning of potential blindness was scary enough, but more illness and possible death? Meeting him was the catalyst I needed to tell my wife that I was getting off all of the prescription drugs and cutting off further treatment. It didn't matter to me if the medication was, in fact, the direct cause of this man's wife dying. Her story set waves of messages through my body, telling me there was no way in hell I was going to take these types of risks.

"I'm going to explore new ways of healing." When I told my wife I would forego Western medicine, it was the first time I felt mentally and intuitively strong enough to say no to what others were imposing upon me.

Traditionally trained as an oncology nurse, she thought I was having a midlife crisis and tried to convince me to continue the traditional route despite my stating my decision was final. I ignored her constant attempts to coerce me back into the system. Her mother was just diagnosed with an aggressive form of cancer, and she was probably afraid of losing us both. Still, I had made up my mind. It wasn't that I was resisting her. I just knew, without a doubt, that I needed to seek alternative methods of healing, while simultaneously having no idea what that meant. This was the beginning of the unraveling of our marriage.

As I looked into alternative treatments, someone suggested I visit a clinic in Switzerland. Serendipitously, on a business trip to Paris, I contacted the doctor, and even though there was usually a six-month wait, there happened to be an opening the week before I left to fly back home to the US. For the first time since searching for effective treatments, I felt heard and understood, and the events that unfolded would forever change my life.

Diagnosing me with heavy metal toxicity, environmental toxins, and a food allergy, the doctor recommended chelation therapy, an expensive, time-consuming procedure that is effective in removing heavy metals from the body.[18] Approaching chelation came with preparation before I traveled back to Europe and underwent the first round of treatment. After that, because I wanted to find care closer to home, I found a doctor in Arizona, but the outcomes weren't as positive as they were after the first round. I concluded that the effectiveness of the treatment I received from the Swiss doc was likely linked to the fact that the therapy is of European origin, created by a German chemist in the 1930s.

After World War II, chelation therapy was used to treat workers who had painted United States naval vessels with lead-based paints. The therapy has been accepted in the US, but it is not easy to access. Because the Food and Drug Administration (FDA) in the United States approved chelation therapy for only a few uses, there are differences in the protocol. My integrative Swiss doc's approach included an emphasis on diet, exercise, and unblocking emotional pathways. He even directed me to have the amalgam fillings in my teeth removed to reduce my mercury exposure.

I found it especially comforting to share that I was doing chelation therapy with my Swiss friends and family. They didn't find it strange or "out there," unlike my American friends. I chose to go to the illogical alternative spaces instead of popping a pill. The pills weren't able to strip away the emotional, mental, spiritual, and physical blockades that prevented me from being pain-free. By the end of that year, the symptoms of my mystery illness had improved dramatically.

While on the mend, my newfound existential explorations began to freak out my wife. "Please don't burn sage at the table. You need to go outside to do that." My wife tolerated my visits to the crystal store, but I was banned from burning sage in the house.

As I questioned my happiness, I often thought about the decision I made to turn down a job as a cruise ship sound engineer—a role that would have taken me around the world—just before our first child was born. Good fathers didn't do that, and anyway, that lifestyle was not complementary to providing children with a healthy upbringing. I didn't regret turning down the position, but I wondered if I could have found a middle ground or looked for a different position somewhere else as a sound engineer. Instead, I changed out of my black t-shirt into a button-down and traded my backstage pass for an employee badge that would get me past the security checkpoint of my office building every morning. At the same time every day, I left home for eight hours to fulfill my duties and provide financially for my family. I was pitifully predictable.

Now, I was loudly and proudly exploring my midlife spiritual awakening.

The Death of Who I Was

Solving the mystery of what was plaguing me by identifying that I had formed a food allergy and was overexposed to environmental toxins and heavy metals meant that I would get to explore the power of the illogical spaces further. Finally, I got the support, understanding, and compassion I needed to heal from the people who were treating my autoimmune disease. My home life, however, remained a different story.

As my spiritual practice grew, my wife and I grew even further apart. I tried to accept that the changes I made were unfamiliar and uncomfortable for her, and adhered as best as I could to the boundaries she imposed upon my transformation. She did her best, too; we were simply moving in different directions. We stopped growing together. We moved into separate bedrooms. As my higher self came alive, the person she expected me to be died.

Like the frustration I felt from the lack of confidence the doctors gave me as I went through the healthcare system, the dynamic of my marriage left both of us feeling alone due to mutual distrust. Feeling like she trusted the doctors more than me, thinking their "best guess" was better than my inner knowledge, I felt angry at her and full of rage toward Western medicine. To heal, I had to transform those emotions. I decided to leave our marriage and open myself up to the limitlessness of my heart.

While our differences of opinion regarding medical attention were the catalyst for our separation, we had years of marital unrest and conflict that had compounded. We recognized that we were no longer growing together, and agreed to divorce amicably.

READER REFLECTION: THE DECONDITIONING OF LOVE

As it stands today, what demands or expectations do you feel you need to meet and fulfill to be loved (in all areas of your life)?

In working to meet those demands and fulfill those expectations, what high-vibe parts of yourself have you left behind (in all areas of your life)?

How can you begin to incorporate sides of yourself that you have been hiding or compartmentalizing because you fear you may not be loved if you show them?

What would it feel like to leave the roles you play behind and show up as your highest vibrational self?

ACTIONABLE INSIGHTS TO HEAL ACROSS FOUR DIMENSIONS OF HEALTH

Emotional

Releasing the need for external validation and practicing self-love enables you to build more authentic and fulfilling connections.

Mental

Challenging the false beliefs and expectations that have shaped your relationships and taking ownership of how you show up in them allows you to reclaim your personal power and live in alignment with your true self.

Physical

Listening to your body's signals and seeking holistic healing methods that address the root causes of your physical discomfort is a long-term solution rather than just treating the symptoms.

Spiritual

Embracing your intuition and exploring new, non-traditional ways of healing and living expands your capacity for spiritual growth and transformation.

SPIRITED ACT OF AUTHENTICITY: THE ART OF SMUDGING—RELEASING LOW VIBES AND INVITING HIGH VIBES

Smudging is an ancient technique used by our ancestors as far back as the Stone Age, and is used today in all cultural circles worldwide. In ancient times, smudging was also used to send sacred messages to the gods. During medieval times, it was used to fend off disease and pandemics, to protect from black magic, and to disinfect a room where a sick patient or family member lay. For thousands of years, people have sought out fragrant and aromatic ingredients like frankincense, spending fortunes to obtain them. This pursuit led to the creation of the ancient Spice Route, a trade route between Asia and Europe.

"What is smudging?" you might ask. To smudge in today's world means using aromatic substances from the plant world, mostly in dry form, and letting them burn over a source of heat, such as a candle or a piece of charcoal, in a fireproof bowl. This is used to cleanse rooms from negative energies and/or to clean our aura or energetic bodies from everyday stressors. In this busy world, we encounter a wide range of spaces and people, each filled with varying, sometimes negative energies. Smudging is then used to clear a space, object, or person from these energies.

When something negative has been removed, I recommend inviting something positive and pure back into the space. Women in ancient Egypt are believed to have smudged a bedroom with wonderful blends made from sandalwood, vetiver, styrax resin, patchouli, and rose. This was believed to stimulate eroticism and sensuality. Some say the men didn't like the smell but succumbed to it once they knew why it was used.

The most popular smudge sticks in the Western world today are made from white sage and palo santo. Other lesser-known plants used are cedar, sweet grass, and yerba santa.

In this Spirited Act of Authenticity, I will teach you how to properly smudge yourself and/or a space.

- Use a fireproof bowl (it should be made of natural materials, such as pottery or soapstone). Indigenous people often use an abalone shell to bring in an element of water. I use a handmade pottery bowl from a local potter (or one I made myself), the smudge stick, or an abalone shell (perfect for loose white sage leaves).

- You will need a feather big enough to gracefully wave the rising smoke in each corner of the room and/or to cover your entire body.

- You should use matches rather than a gas lighter, creating a different, gentler energy. I use the long firestarter matches (11 inches) for this, so I don't burn my fingers.

People Clearing

- Have your fireproof bowl or abalone shell ready. Light your match and hold it in your dominant hand. Take your smudge stick, hold it in your less dominant hand (for right-handed people, use your left hand), and light the front of the smudge stick for about 20-30 seconds. You should have a nice smoke going.

- Now, blow out the match, place it in a safe container, and move the smudge stick like a wand around your entire body, swirling it over your limbs and trunk until you sense that all negative energy is gone. You can also use a feather.

- Speak your intentions or prayer while moving the smudge stick over your body. One of the most beautiful prayers I use when smudging myself, which I've learned from our Indigenous people.

May your hands be cleansed, that they create beautiful things.

May your feet be cleansed, that they might take you where you most need to be.

May your heart be cleansed, that you might hear its messages clearly.

May your throat be cleansed, that you might speak rightly when words are needed.

May your eyes be cleansed, that you might see the signs and wonders of the world.

May this person and space be washed clean by the smoke of these fragrant plants.

And may that same smoke carry our prayers, spiraling, to the heavens.

- Once finished, put the smudge stick in a fireproof bowl or dish, such as an Abalone shell, and let it extinguish naturally. The smudge should stop after a few minutes.

- Please be careful and never leave it unattended. It's a good time to sit in silence and reflect, and wait for the process and smudge to subside naturally.

Object Clearing

- I use a fireproof bowl, fill it three-quarters full with sand, and then light a charcoal tablet, like the ones used for incense burning or a hookah. Use metal tongs to light the charcoal until it starts to spark. Place the charcoal tablet on top of the sand and wait until the tablet turns from black to gray. Please be careful not to do this near flammable objects such as curtains, tablecloths, or paper!

- Now, sprinkle the top of your charcoal with your favorite smudge blend. Of course, you can also use an abalone shell without a charcoal tablet. Just light your white sage stick and lay it on top. Be careful—this gets hot too, so please don't burn yourself!

- Now, you are ready to smudge your apartment or house. You can find various instructions online. Some people suggest going from the front door through the house and then coming back. Some say you must go clockwise to achieve the desired effect. I believe there are no specific rules, as your intention matters more. That said, I have found in my practice that the most effective way to cleanse a space is to follow this general guide.

- Close all windows and doors except for your front door.

- Starting from the top floor, go through each room counterclockwise, fanning the smoke into each corner. Pay particular attention to areas that feel heavy or dark, and wave some more smudges in that direction.

- Move down to the next floor until you reach your front door. Calmly yet resolutely fan the energies out through the door. If you have a basement, proceed there next. Move through each area counterclockwise, sweeping the energies up and out through the front door.

- There are some nice prayers you can use before you enter each room or when you start your ritual. I suggest this one, but you can also come up with your own.

> *"May all darkness disappear; may only love and light now reappear."*

- Once you are done, leave the front door open for a few minutes. You could go through each room again with a rattle or a drum to enhance the clearing. Follow your intuition.

- At this stage, I suggest you go through the entire house again, but this time in a clockwise direction.

I use my fireproof bowl with a sweeter scent, such as Kyphi or King David's Temptation. You can find some amazing smudge blends from various small businesses on Etsy, or mix your own. Again, there are no rules; just use your imagination and have fun experimenting.

Sacred Scribbles *(Use these pages as a portal for decoding visions, tracking soul whispers, or just letting the ink remember what your heart already knows.)*

5

SELF-LOVE THROUGH AFFIRMATION: INVITING DIVINE INTERVENTION

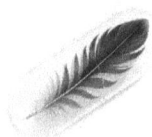

O ne act of self-love, saying no to continuing down the road of Western medicine treatments, led me to a second act, releasing myself from a marriage that no longer aligned with who we each had become in our middle adulthood. It turns out that emotions are contagious. Love is no exception. Each act of self-love created a positive ripple effect that would help me move past the pain and loneliness that I encountered in the years following the divorce. My feedback systems were elevating in vibration, yet I knew there was so much more I had to confront, especially concerning love.

I moved out of the house I shared with my wife in the spring after we decided to end our marriage. To support myself through the transition, I signed up for a retreat with medical anthropologist Alberto Villoldo of The Four Winds Society and traveled to Germany for my first round of chelation therapy.[19] Grieving the end of my marriage and figuring out how to manage the dispersal of my family, while I knew it was the right thing for all of us, felt sad and, at times, uncomfortable.

Amid my post-divorce heartache, I came to see that what had made me sick were layers of physical, mental, emotional, and spiritual toxins and stressors that were stored in the trillions of cells that make up my body. There were also positive indicators that provided me with evidence, increasing my confidence in using my intuition in decision-making.

I increasingly paid more attention to the positive aspects of my past, as I reframed negative situations to help me understand my behaviors. Looking back on my childhood, I recall the unity and safety I felt on those Sunday mornings with my mom, dad, and siblings. I decided that I would recreate those feelings as an adult. How could I do that alone? My kids were becoming adults now, and while we spent time together, most often the only warm body filling the house was mine. While figuring out the new dynamics that came with solo living, I invested in working to design a new Sunday routine of solitude, and continued to relieve the remaining symptoms I had from my mystery illness by furthering the exploration of more illogical spaces.

The day I told my wife I was going to look for alternative ways to heal, I had never heard of Energy Medicine. I considered energy as nothing more than the fuel you need for a workout. It was through the Grow a New Body Retreat that I was introduced to Energy Medicine, resetting my physical health by nourishing my body with specific neuro-nutrients and superfoods.[20] In combination with healing modalities that ranged from yoga to ceremonial rituals and oxygen therapy, I was happily immersed in the world of the illogical. Funnily enough, it all made perfect sense to me, as did the chelation therapy treatments I underwent. Imagine a river and its tributaries filled with garbage or toxic waste flowing through your body. That's what was happening in mine. The chelation therapy essentially acted like a magnet that could pick up the trash and remove it from my system.

Energy Medicine is an extensively used term, likely of Chinese origin, but there is some information suggesting that it originated in Japan. The Eastern teachings made their mark on the Western world when four researchers gathered in Boulder, Colorado, in the late 1980s and coined the term.[21] Thousands of years ago, Chinese healers identified twelve major energetic pathways in the body that make up a complex web that links the limbs and organs together.[22] The inner and outer workings of our bodies are connected by energetic streams flowing into and away from one another. Acupuncture, Reiki, and Chakra Balancing are forms of Energy Medicine.

High-Vibe Nourishment[IP]

The composition of life is cellular. In the first hours after conception, we are one cell. After three days, we are two. From there, our cellular makeup multiplies. A newborn brain contains more than 100 billion brain cells.[23] An adult has exponentially more cells, the number so large that it will not fit on this page. Cells need energy to survive, which they gain from food, molecules, or sunlight. Because of this, you may have heard people say, "Everything is energy."

My natural first step was to begin using food as medicine, providing my body with the nourishment it needs to regenerate itself. The environmental and heavy metal toxicity that had built up in my cellular makeup throughout my life was systematically removed through chelation therapy. To back up that work, I found it beneficial to start creating a new relationship with food, drink, and my body image. My work at the retreat helped me understand how good it felt to nourish my body with whole, organic foods. By eliminating caffeine, alcohol, meat, and dairy, I was able to conduct my private mini-experiment, connecting what I excluded and included in my diet to how I felt emotionally, mentally, and physically. While excluding different food groups and beverages was sustainable for the duration of the retreat, it was not a way of living that I wanted to maintain. I did not want to live without the joy that comes to me through cooking delicious meals, eating a wide variety of foods, and appreciating wine or bourbon, especially in the company of close friends.

When I paid close attention to the feelings that would arise when I was eating and drinking, I realized that underneath the enjoyment was a lot of negative self-talk. I was judging my food harshly and telling myself a lot of negative stories about my body. Having been fixated on my desire to lose weight, I realized that how I spoke to myself about food was the real problem. I needed to shed the unhealthy dialogue. Taking the learnings from the Grow a New Body Retreat and the other teachers I worked with, going forward, I decided that I was ready to use food as medicine and relate to it in healthier ways that I could maintain for the long haul. A high-vibe response system was forming in the physical dimension of my health due to making choices based on how I wanted to feel rather than how I didn't want to feel.

Before, during, and after eating fresh summer peaches with Burrata, I felt great from head to toe. Before, during, and after eating Chinese takeout, I felt a bit guilty, unfulfilled, swollen, and upset in my stomach. This wasn't a judgment call on the food. It is about how our self-judgments energetically connect with it. It's not about good or bad; it is about paying attention to my intention with what I am putting into my body.

Low- or high-vibrational energy directly relates to the outcomes of our choices and habits of consumption. Noticing that I began some of my meals in the same way I approached eating Chinese takeout, with guilt and emotional emptiness, changed the course of my actions. Ninety-five percent of what I eat is high-vibrational by nature. Meaning that much of my diet is centered on colorful vegetables from the farmers' market, a little organic protein, and other whole foods. The other five percent might be a breakfast sandwich from my favorite coffee chain when I am on the road, or an evening when I decide to order pizza and watch a movie. Before I understood the impact my energy had on what I eat and how I eat it, I placed judgment on myself. Shaming myself for having some French fries, for instance, I now understand that it is more damaging to myself than if I focus on the energy that I bring to my meals, no matter what I am eating.

No, I am not saying that if my diet consisted of highly processed foods and takeout meals, my high-vibrational energy alone would make me healthy. Connecting the dots between the logical and illogical has helped me embrace the reality that moderating portions, tuning into my fullness levels by eating mindfully, eating a diet rich in whole or minimally processed foods, and allowing myself to enjoy and indulge within reason keeps me emotionally, mentally, physically, and spiritually healthy.

Both restriction and over-consumption are low-vibrational behaviors for me. Moderation allows me to savor and fully enjoy not only the food I am eating or the wine I am appreciating, but also the company that surrounds me. To me, that is a form of deconditioning myself from self-loathing. To receive the love I have for myself, I have to be a guy who respects his body. The depth of love I can receive socially and relationally around the table increases because I am no longer distracted by the low-vibrational energies I had formed around food and my body. When we sit down to a meal with a feeling of low self-worth, we miss out on the love in and around us.

We all have a direct line to what nourishes our body by transforming our energy from low to high vibe and experimenting with how our health responds. Personally, I didn't want to eliminate the five percent of my diet that allows for some freedom to eat a piece of cake. Everyone is different, and your approach will be unique to you. I strongly believe that the patterns and belief systems we have formed around consumption are what's behind our dis-ease.

Beginning with the energetic vibrational exchanges we have with what's on our plate and in our glass is a great way to begin forming new and healthy habits that heal from the inside out. The decisions I made in support of feeling great have released me from loads of bad information and false conditioning that held me back from self-love.

As a man, I realized that my low-vibe relationship with food was shaped by what I was taught about openly discussing diet, exercise, and body image. Many societal and cultural constructs had told me that I needed to do things like go on a carnivore diet or develop a six-pack. Expressing insecurities was not a part of male nutrition programs, or at least none I could find at the time. Creating a high vibe relationship with myself meant I had to stop engaging with the outside world, be present at the table, and be kind to my body, which had gotten me through so much. The movement of energy in and out of my system took on a much deeper meaning beyond the amount of calories I ate and the extent to which I moved my body.

The Art of Passive Healing

The first time I felt energy in my body was during a "Despacho Ceremony" at the Grow a New Body Retreat in Europe. In the ceremony, a prayer bundle is created to offer to Mother Earth. It is typically made of flowers, seeds, things found in nature, candies, and even white sugar, symbolizing sweetness and love. There are no rules for what is included in the offering. Participants can contribute personally, including photos or a page from their journal. Everyone sets their intentions and contributes their prayer to the bundle before it is wrapped up and buried, burned, or placed into running water. Ultimately, it is an expression of love and appreciation for Mother Earth. The specific Despacho we did that day is called Ainy Despacho. Ainy, which is Quechuan for "Right Relations," invites us to align our lives by forming intimate connections with others in all facets of our lives (job, family, friends, etc.). Moving through the loss of my marriage, immersed in a stressful corporate career while excitedly building my new life, the ceremony was an unexpected remedy that helped me bridge the gap between sorrow and renewal.

Standing amidst the ruins of a castle on the borders of Switzerland, Germany, and France during the ceremony, I raised my right hand in the air to give thanks, and I felt energy hit my hand for the first time. It felt like a pressure washer hitting my palm. Startled and unsure what to make of it, I asked Alberto about it after the ceremony.

"You must develop that," he said and walked away.

"How do I do that?" I wondered.

While the illogical spaces I was exploring were helping me heal, I never considered taking on a professional role in the healing arts. I was a novice in a new space. So, what was I to do with this crazy sensation in my hands?

After the retreat, I told my friend Jeff about what had happened. He had much more experience in the realm of alternative medicine. "You should do Reiki," he told me.

I thought he was crazy for saying this. "Me?" I barely understood what Reiki was, but there was a knowing inside of me that he was right. I was an executive at a bank. There was no way I could perform Reiki; I knew if I did that, my reality would crumble.

In the Fall of that year, my divorce was final, and I had made significant improvements to my health. The chronic pain paled in intensity, and I even had moments of feeling pain-free. As the new year began, my pain came to an end. I was healed.

Jeff's recommendation that I become a Reiki Practitioner lingered in my mind after the retreat. As I recalled the past, I realized that I had not fully shown up in relationships because I was carrying around that little backpack I wore on the walk to school and back every day, filled with fear of being hurt. Identifying this was helpful. Heartbroken, I was ready to love again.

Reiki is the art of passive healing. It is the ability to feel energy, the awareness of the vibration of the energy, and the identification of where the body may have an imbalance. Like Beatrix's mother resting her hands on her daughter's blue bruises (see Chapter 3), it's an intentional healing modality based purely on energy flow from one person to another. You do not go in and remove anything. Instead, you assist by helping shift and move the energy through the body. It is a form of guiding energy through gentle touch and hovering the hands over the body.

After I shared that I was still struggling with loneliness and isolation post-divorce, a good friend suggested I check out Louise Hay's Affirmations for Self-Healing.[24] I quickly took her advice.

"I love myself. I approve of myself." For 60 days straight, I practiced my first affirmation. "I love myself. I approve of myself." I parked a 5-minute walk from my office door, allowing me to use the time to recite my affirmations out loud or visualize them between 30 and 60 times each day. On day 61 of using these affirmations, a sudden feeling of bliss washed over me. I felt an overwhelming sense of acceptance and unconditional love for myself. This whole affirmation thing was working. I was ready to take Jeff's advice to become a Reiki Practitioner.

I signed up for training and became a Certified Reiki Master, the highest level of training available, only one year after my divorce was finalized. I was taking my health into my own hands, and I could begin to help others. It became apparent that the deeper I dove into my healing, the happier I would become. A new way of life was forming, and now that included a new line of work that I considered a side passion project to counteract the stress of my day job. I started my private healing practice, but kept it hidden. If people at work only knew that I was getting involved with this work, I thought they would think I had lost my mind and never speak to me again.

We Need You

Continuing the work that I had done on my relationship with food and my body, the year after I completed Reiki Certification, I was introduced to the work of the International Council of Thirteen Indigenous Grandmothers.[25] A group of Indigenous elder women allied to share their ancient cultures and traditions, ensuring the knowledge of their tribes could be spread and preserved in the name of "Reverence for All Creation." I discovered that the Grandmothers were gathering in Sedona, Arizona, close to my home in Scottsdale, and signed up to participate. Like every other illogical experiment, I went with an open mind without a clue as to what would come from the experience.

Grandmother Rita Pitka Blumenstein was the first person in Alaska certified as a traditional doctor of medicine and the first non-medical doctor to serve at the Alaska Native Hospital. Recognized from childhood for her healing gifts, she helped deliver babies and cared for the sick long before she was formally honored. Guided by the teachings of her grand-mothers and great-grandmothers, she became a visionary elder whose wisdom bridged generations. Her life was devoted to healing, resilience, and reminding us that we are here for the universe, not just ourselves. At the opening ceremony of the Grandmother's Gathering, I witnessed her sitting on a blanket on the stone floor, wearing an ankle-length black dress and furry slippers. Playing a handheld drum made out of moose hide, painted with colorful Yup'ik symbols, her crescent moon smile and infectious, high-toned laughter complemented the beat. I decided to approach her and introduce myself.

Before I knew it, I was next to her. She reached out and took my head between her hands. Deep rivers of wisdom were carved out of the corners of her eye, moving upstream, circulating her forehead, and downstream, gracing the length of her face. Joy flowed out of her open mouth. "We need you. We need you. We need you. Don't be afraid," she looked me directly in the eyes, an act of love I had not experienced since I was a small child. "Don't be afraid. Don't be afraid," she said as she held my head between her hands and delicately blew her breath into my third eye. "You will be able to puncture nasty boils filled with pus with your fingers." Her voice was quiet and clear, with the sweet tone of a whimsical narrator you meet in cinematic dream sequences.

My hands began to vibrate subtly. On the surface, her message sounded funny, signaling that I had hidden superpowers as a master pimple-popper. Still, I did not get lost in the translation or my tendency to use humor in serious situations. Her words were an intensely comforting warning. Something gross, maybe even terrible, would be coming my way, and I could heal it with my hands.

When an Indigenous person blows their breath into your third eye, it is often a sacred act that carries deep spiritual significance. The **third eye**, located between the eyebrows, is considered in many traditions to be the center of intuition, insight, and spiritual vision. By blowing breath onto this area, the Indigenous healer or spiritual guide may be engaging in a form of energy transfer or blessing, intended to activate or awaken your third eye, connect you to spiritual realms, or clear any blockages in your intuitive and spiritual pathways.

In many Indigenous cultures, breath is considered a powerful life force, often referred to as prana in Indian traditions, or similar concepts in other spiritual practices. Blowing breath may symbolize the giving of life, energy, or spiritual wisdom from one person to another. The act could also be seen as a way to help you align with your higher self, deepen your connection with the earth, or open your awareness to spiritual insights.

The meaning behind the gesture may vary depending on the specific cultural tradition and the intention of the person performing it, but overall, it is likely a deeply respectful, sacred, and healing act.

When I put "Reiki Master" on my public digital media platforms, I thought the world was going to end. But it was time to be my authentic self with all of my gifts. I was ready to brush off the critics, but they never came forward. Instead, I had more meaningful conversations, and people contacted me to ask questions and share stories that had similarities with mine.

I was honored that Grandmother Rita recognized the healing energy in my hands. Her premonition that something more was coming made me wonder what more I could handle. I was finally healed. Or was I? Whatever was coming, I felt a trust in something far more significant than myself that helped me find a sense of security through the fear. I knew I would be sent more existential guideposts, but this time, I understood I wouldn't have to confront them alone.

READER REFLECTION: THE VIBRATION OF SELF-LOVE

When it comes to your relationships with people, consumption, and your body, where are some areas where you are experiencing low-vibrational energy?

When it comes to your relationships with other people, consumption, and your body, where are some areas where you are experiencing high-vibrational energy?

What would your life be like if you transformed the relationships in your life from low- to high-vibrational?

What is one small act of self-love you can take to begin to vibe higher?

ACTIONABLE INSIGHTS TO HEAL ACROSS FOUR DIMENSIONS OF HEALTH

Emotional

Releasing past resentment and embracing self-love allows you to heal emotional wounds and create space for positive growth.

Mental

Reframing negative self-talk and internal judgments empowers you to build a healthier relationship with yourself and others.

Physical

Using food as medicine and becoming mindful of the energy surrounding your eating habits can lead to better physical health and well-being.

Spiritual

Trusting in your intuition and engaging in spiritual practices that resonate with you opens you up to deeper healing and spiritual connection.

SPIRITED ACT OF AUTHENTICITY: SUNDAY MORNING RITUAL AND SELF-LOVE MEDITATION

I love Sunday mornings. Probably because a leisurely, late breakfast with lots of yummy foods was celebrated and cherished growing up in my family. To this day, I make it a point to light candles and play classical music. I turn off my phone and reflect on my week. Sometimes, I draw an oracle card or just admire nature outside. This is a time to take it slow and check in with myself—mind/body/soul. What do I need today and this week? I often hear a gentle whisper now and then to take a salt bath, find a new hike with Lili (my Aussiedoodle canine companion), or just sit and read a book. I love the rainy days the most, as they give me an excuse to stay in, curl up, and do some self-care.

Here are some of my suggestions to create a relaxing Sunday morning for yourself:

- Buy a nice candle candelabra, set it in the middle of your dining table, and light candles. I sometimes have so many candles in various places and shapes that it creates an environment like Christmas. Those of you who've been to Europe during Christmas and experienced the coziness of that season know what I mean.

- Find your favorite classical music station or stream it with your favorite service. There are so many great playlists there. I suggest something from the Baroque epoch, as scientific experiments have proven that Baroque music improves focus, lowers stress and anxiety, and can contribute to emotional resilience.

- Brew your favorite tea or make a yummy latte.

- Try to turn off your cell phone for 4–6 hours.

- I fix a typical Swiss breakfast, which consists of Zopf Bread (like Challah Bread), grass-fed butter, homemade jams, and some yogurt. You can see that this might not necessarily reflect the healthy lifestyle that you're expecting me to preach. One of my best friends is a pastry chef and health coach. She often reminds me that what initially seems like an oxymoron is her philosophy of creating healthier versions of your favorite foods and eating them in moderation.

If you think your food is wholesome and nourishing, you can also have what might look like something (un) healthy and not worry about it. Kind of tricking your mind. If you think something is bad for you, it's creating a negative vibration and is probably bad for you. If you tell yourself that this piece of pie is good for you and will make you feel amazing, then that is what your cells will receive as a positive signal.

This doesn't mean that I think it's healthy to overeat sugar. It is about creating a new conversation between you and food that won't leave you feeling guilty and ashamed. That will only leave you stressed and perpetuate a low vibe. It's a mindset, and again, I just treat myself on Sundays as a way to relax and feel better while still nourishing myself.

- Read a book, take a bath, and check in with yourself.

- What do YOU need today? Take a break from serving or pleasing others for a few hours. Make Sunday *your* day.

- As a special treat, I am gifting you this special self-love meditation I've recorded. Find a comfortable space to lie down, put on some headphones, and immerse yourself in this high-vibe recording. Just scan the QR code to get access.

Sacred Scribbles *(Use these pages as a portal for decoding visions, tracking soul whispers, or just letting the ink remember what your heart already knows.)*

6

BONDS THAT DON'T BREAK: FEELING SAFE IN THE UNKNOWN

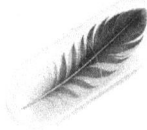

When my wife was nine months pregnant with our second child, we moved our family to Eagle River, Alaska. I was offered a promotion, provided I was willing to relocate. My supervisor saw potential in my abilities and invited me to be part of a management training program. One of the facilitators advised us that to get ahead in the company, one should consider a job nobody wanted. When a managerial role in Anchorage was posted on the corporate intranet, this was the perfect opportunity for me to do exactly that. Apply for a job that nobody else wants. The job offer came six weeks later.

When I broke the news to my wife, the stress sent her into labor. Alaska is a place of extremes, with only a few hours of sunlight in the winter and only a few hours of darkness in the summer. We never anticipated settling down there. After some deliberation, we saw the promotion as a great financial opportunity for our family, and I accepted the job.

When we were dating early on, it was established that neither of us wanted to get married or have children. I always say that my daughter was on a mission to be born. It turned out that the decision on whether to have a family wasn't entirely up to us or birth control. When we went to the hospital for the first ultrasound, we entered as two people who were nervous and reluctant to be parents. Hearing my daughter's heartbeat and seeing her little body forming on the screen, I was ecstatic and fell in love immediately. Those cliché ultrasound scenes we see in the movies are true to life. Anticipating her arrival, I couldn't stop thinking about preparing for the moment we would meet. When my daughter was born and I held her for the first time, our love was permanently embedded in my body. When my son was conceived, it was no different, except that I had about four years of parenting experience.

My son was six weeks old when we moved to Alaska. This was when my wife and I had different work schedules. She worked as a nurse, mostly in the mornings from eight until noon, and I worked the afternoon and night shifts from one to ten. That meant I would watch the kids in the early part of the day, and she would take care of them in the afternoons and evenings. Caring for two kids under five was a bit of a challenge, but the moments I would zip them up in their snowsuits, seeing their cute little faces, warm and cozy, made it all worth it. My son had the cutest little button nose. In the tiniest moments, when I was alone with them, I would feel the same connective bond I had felt when seeing them on the ultrasound screen.

In Alaska, earthquakes occur often. On average, there are fifty to one hundred quakes daily, accounting for more than half of the earthquakes in the United States.[26] There are roughly half a dozen at a magnitude of six or more on the Richter Scale, an average of forty-five between five and six, and over three hundred between four and five. Moving to Alaska, one of the first things you learn is the recommended safety guidelines when a tremor strikes. One of the recommendations at the time was to stand in a doorway.

One morning, a quake around five on the Richter Scale started. The kids were close to me; as luck would have it, we were near a door frame. I pulled them against me, and the three of us stood out the quake together. Standing there, I felt confident that I was protecting them. The doorway was safe because that's what I was told. As parents, we do everything we can to keep our children safe. Often, we rely on information from other parents, government agencies, teachers, and medical professionals because they are experts and specialists. We learn as we go; winging it a bit and relying on outside information helps us "hack" parenting with the tips and tricks that have worked for others or the tried methods tested in a lab.

As my kids grew, I signed up to be the dad who would coach their soccer teams, cheer them on, watch as they scored, and give them a pep talk when they didn't. As they became teenagers, we navigated a period when their brains were developing the capacity for reasoning, but not yet mature enough to make the most informed decisions. There were arguments, yelling, and sometimes screaming. While there were flashes of wanting to walk away, there was a knowing that I would see them through the entirety of their life.

As they grew into adults, our relationship felt more like we were on equal footing; the conversations became more complex, and I realized the impact of my decisions on them. When conflict arose between us, I experienced my wounds from my childhood creeping in. My face would turn red, and my hands would tremble. I felt guilty for losing my cool and accepted that no matter how old they were, I was obligated to communicate carefully with my kids, rather than acting like a child myself.

We have had rifts to repair, and I have seen it as my role to be consistent and encouraging in telling them that there is nothing we cannot mend together. When they moved away from home and started their adult life, there was an acceptance of letting go that I had to contend with and make peace with. I could no longer provide them with a protective doorway during scary times.

Crossing Thresholds

It turns out that standing in the doorway during an earthquake is one of the worst and most dangerous places to be.[27] The recommendation has now not only been disproved but also warned against. It is now understood that doorways may not structurally support the building or protect it from collapsing. They may even be weaker than the walls. The thing about requirements, recommendations, and information proven through scientific studies and research is that the conclusions evolve.

This isn't to say that everything we're told is false or harmful. The best scientists in the world keep asking questions, that's why information often evolves and, at times, seems conflicting. It is safe to say that everything is an experiment, and the information we are provided is often presented as "logical spaces" because of the depth of testing to prove a hypothesis correct or incorrect, and the societal, governmental, and cultural credibility behind the source of information. In the case of an earthquake, if the government of Alaska recommends a safety measure, I learned to automatically trust that it was the best way to protect my kids. If I had conducted my experiment by asking questions from both the "logical" and "illogical" spaces," I might have devised an alternative to the doorway. That information could have stemmed from examining our home's structure, noting the frame's thinness, and realizing we could be vulnerable to debris, or it might have come from my research, which could have involved finding alternative locations that seemed more sensible to me.

We think that we are keeping our children safe by following the orders of the land, when the orders of the land are orchestrated by other humans who are seeking the answers too. Every bit of information we give and receive is subject to change. When we wrap our minds around this, the mechanisms of control we use to keep each other safe can be released. In that headspace, we can find comfort in the unknown, which helps bring us back to the high-vibrational responsiveness of the unconditional heartspace.

When my wife did not want me to stop the Western treatments for my mystery illness, she thought it was best for me because that is what she was taught. Her mother was diagnosed with cancer around the same time. Faced with family members who are sick, we often become scared of anything that could potentially treat dis-ease outside of the systems that are most prevalently recommended.

Nearly twenty years after having stood with the kids in the doorway, I was diagnosed with non-Hodgkin lymphoma. There I was, walking out of the doorway of another hospital. Cancer. I had cancer. Only ten days before my oncologist told me the news, I crossed the threshold of another doorway into a new home. I was out of the corporate apartment, ready to start my life again.

The news that I had cancer came after being misdiagnosed twice; the first time with strep throat, and the second with a regrown tonsil. Having gone through the frustrations of treating my autoimmune disease, I was even more frustrated with Western medicine. Finally, biopsies were taken that revealed that the lump that had formed in the back of my throat was cancer. As much as I hated the outcome, for the first time, I had a clear diagnosis.

Even though Grandmother Rita Pitka Blumenstein had warned me that something was coming, I did not expect that the boils she was referencing would metastasize into cancer. My reaction was one of quiet panic. After receiving the news in the middle of the societal lockdown during a global pandemic,

I returned home to ask "Dr. Search Engine" some questions. What was the life expectancy of a middle-aged man with non-Hodgkin lymphoma? How do I tell my kids I have cancer? What is the cure? Will I need chemotherapy? Some of the answers and advice that came up scared me, but ultimately, I learned that the survival rate was high, and found slivers of gratitude that I had one of "the best types of cancer." I calmed down in preparation to share the news with my kids.

Knowing that I had become increasingly well-educated and trained in the healing arts and Energy Medicine and disheartened by Western medicine, my kids begged me to follow through with my oncologist's recommendations, including chemotherapy. Facing them, I knew they wanted to keep me safe. I wanted them to know I would do anything to stay alive. I agreed to stand under the doorway again, not knowing my destiny, but this time, I would not leave my health up to only the logical spaces.

I decided to use everything I had learned and go even deeper into the illogical spaces to get to the root of why I was sick again, and why this time it was cancer. Having pummeled through work while going through my mystery illness, I made a courageous decision to take a medical leave of absence. Assuring my boss that I would be back was incredibly scary for me. I was in the latter stages of leading the development of a product set up to dramatically change how we did business for the better. Worried that taking time to heal would be a sign of weakness in the corporate world, I was confident I could recover quickly and return to work swiftly. I used the time to continue seeing my oncologist and began seeking additional care from an integrative doctor in Germany.

That wasn't all. I employed psychic mediums and intuitives to help me understand things like karmic soul plans, and used past-life regression to open up the spiritual aspect of what was cursing my health. Faced with potential death, I decided that nothing was off-limits. I saw everything I tried as a possible cure. Insecurities from my childhood continued to rise within me, and I had the opportunity to pay attention to the messages and training that helped me understand I could rewrite my relationship with life's experiences.

Flawsome[IP]

I lost my hair, and my body was swollen from the chemotherapy, much more than after I ate Chinese food. Looking at myself was painful, and it brought back the low body image I had developed from feeling rejected as a kid and throughout my attempts to have successful intimate relationships. Sitting in the waiting room to see my oncologist, I never felt like a sick cancer patient. This way of thinking would help me going forward.

I knew that the side effects of the chemotherapy treatments could threaten my mental strength if I didn't take action to create a high vibe for myself. I had to do something to keep myself strong and engaged. Given the positive impact affirmations had on me in the past, I decided to do the Louise Hay Mirror Challenge, a beautiful self-love exercise.[28]

"I love you. I love you. I love you," I would tell myself as I looked into the mirror every day for 21 days. Staring back at me was a 50-year-old man with no hair on my head, no eyebrows, and no beard. Even though I looked like my ex-girlfriend's naked pet guinea pig, tears of compassion for myself and a deep love of who I was at my core would pour down my face.

"I love you. I love you. I love you." While admiring yourself in a mirror might sound simple or even ridiculous, embracing my reflection was one of the hardest and most important things I have ever done. I began to release the notion that I was flawed and even created a new word for myself: flawsome.

Taking lessons from Grandmother Rita, The Four Winds Society, becoming a Reiki Master, and working with the clients of my healing practice, I rocketed forward into furthering my self-discovery. After multiple trips to Germany, four rounds of chemo, using food as medicine, training, learning under the Q'ero shamans of Peru, and working with psychic mediums, my oncologist pronounced that I was in remission less than a year after being diagnosed. I went back to Germany to clear the toxins from the chemo out of my system and returned to work.

"You've been reassigned." On my first day back at the office, I was told that I was permanently pulled off the project I was leading before I left. "We didn't think you would come back."

The words that were spoken to me that day signaled how little my existence was valued at work. Even worse, I wondered if they had considered me dead. I knew it was a risk when I took medical leave to focus on getting better. A colleague of mine had worked full-time through two bouts of cancer, and I witnessed the praise of her "strength" and "resilience." Those words were great ways to describe her. She had gone through so much. The problem, I believe, was that behind the accolades was self-interest on the part of the company.

I suspect that it was likely that she had the same fear I had, worrying about the negative repercussions of taking medical leave. I had decided my health mattered more to me than the potential benefits of staying the course at work, and felt convinced that the company feared losing money more than losing a life. Now here I was, back at work, immersed in a low-vibrational reactionary system. Quietly, I accepted the reassignment, knowing it threatened my self-worth. The work I was doing at the office contradicted my work helping others at my healing practice. I didn't know how to detach from the title I had earned. The one my parents were proud of. The one that helped put my kids through college. The one that had defined me, yet had nothing to do with who I was now becoming.

My life was not yet congruent. A deceptive office in the C-Suite defined my likeness as a corporate executive. This logical space, posing as big and important, was an isolating, standardized, and uninspiring facade. Yes, I had accomplished a lot, but I was now in a position to renegotiate contracts I had made with myself, so I could get off this roller coaster of disease and choose my experiences while I still had a spot here on earth.

READER REFLECTION: EXPLORING THE ILLOGICAL AND LOGICAL SPACES

What are your current fears, dangers, and things you worry about that keep you up at night? (List all that comes to mind.)

Choose one of your answers.

What have you been told, or how do you believe you have been conditioned to create that fear?

What illogical spaces or modalities can you use to treat the root cause of this fear?

How would the way you live your life change if this fear were eliminated?

ACTIONABLE INSIGHTS TO HEAL ACROSS FOUR DIMENSIONS OF HEALTH

Emotional

Releasing the need for external validation and acknowledging your inner strength allows you to find peace and acceptance, even in challenging times.

Mental

Questioning the information you've been given and exploring both logical and illogical spaces empowers you to make decisions that align with your true values.

Physical

Paying attention to your body's signals and taking proactive steps to address your health holistically ensures that you prioritize your well-being over societal expectations.

Spiritual

Trusting in your intuition and participating in spiritual practices that resonate with you allows deeper healing and spiritual growth, even in the face of uncertainty.

SPIRITED ACT OF AUTHENTICITY: HOW TO CREATE A DESPACHO CEREMONY

Despacho Ceremonies have been a part of Peruvian culture for centuries, and are celebrated on various occasions such as birthdays, weddings, and deaths. They are usually celebrated and led by the Laika (high shamans or wisdom keepers of the Q'ero lineage of Peru). Still, the ceremony can also be done as a family ritual or in an individual setting. This specific Despacho is called Ainy Despacho. Ainy is Quechua, speaking about the fact that we're all connected, hence inviting us to bring all of our lives (job, family, friends, etc.) into a right and harmonious relationship. I've learned this from my friends at the Four Winds Society, and I wanted to share it with you, translating it so that you could benefit from this powerful technique, even though it may sound unfamiliar to you. Ultimately, you will feel an energy shift that catapults you into a healing space.

You will need the following "ingredients," all of them biodegradable, please.

- A large, white or brown piece of paper (at least 35x35 inches in diameter)
- Red and white carnations (about a dozen each)
- Leaves from native plants around you, or you can use bay leaves in winter
- One small shell represents the womb of the earth
- Sugar represents the sweetness of life
- Rice or various grains, representing fertility and abundance
- Various grains and rice represent sustenance
- Nuts, representing gifts for the plant people
- Various dried beans, representing protection and abundance
- Corn in various colors, again representing sustenance and a gift back to the Earth for what we have been given
- Raisins, a gift for the spirits of our ancestors, our blood lineage
- Figs: spirits of the ancient ones who dwell in the sacred mountains
- Alphabet noodles represent the ability to step outside and beyond language
- Animal crackers, representing animal spirits and health

One of my teachers loved to add more sweetness to her Despacho ceremony. These are some examples, but feel free to use whatever you have in your pantry or what brings you joy.

- Candies, candy hearts, sweet gum drops, candy corn, etc., represent everything we are in a relationship with
- Chocolate: Pachamama (Mother Earth) LOVES chocolate
- Loose sage or other incense, feeding the elements of the Earth
- Black licorice for protection
- Gummy or candy frogs represent messengers and envoys to carry our prayers
- "Play" money (one piece) to ensure the Despacho's success and bring abundance to your life. (Note: some people use real one-dollar bills.)
- Unraveled cotton balls (clouds), representing awake time and dream time
- Confetti stars, representing our connection to the cosmos
- Colored confetti or sprinkles to celebrate all life
- Rainbow yarn represents the bridge between the worlds (ours and the spirit world, i.e., our ancestors)
- Red and white ribbons to honor our path as humans with a physical body (red like blood) and spiritual nature (white)
- Various flower petals for healing

You are ready to get started.

- Start by placing the large piece of paper on the floor or in the middle of a big table.

- Then, place the shell or a big flower petal in the center of the paper.

- Next, sprinkle some of the sugar all over the paper.

- Now, take the flower petals, leaves, and carnations, and blow your prayers individually into each one. Place them on the piece of paper and start to arrange them in a mandala-like fashion.

- It's time to have fun with it. Use all other ingredients and place them in a geometrical fashion on the paper around the flowers and leaves.

- Sprinkle the extra sweetness, animal crackers, alphabet noodles, money, confetti, sprinkles, etc., onto your Despacho.

- Lay the yarn in a nice pattern across the design.

- Once completed, the Despacho is carefully folded from the outside and wrapped and secured with a ribbon or string. Be careful not to disturb the beautiful pattern. Think of it as a fragile object, and decorate the outside of the pattern with leftover flowers or ribbon.

- The bundle can then be ceremonially buried (for slow, steady results), burned (for quicker transformation), or fed to running waters, thus conveying the gifts to *Spirit*. Again, please use biodegradable materials so we don't add unnecessary waste to Pacha Mama (Mother Earth)!

If the Despacho is burned, someone should stay with the fire until the embers are cold, if possible. Do not put water on the fire. Ashes created in this sacred fire should be buried in the earth at a later time.

Sacred Scribbles *(Use these pages as a portal for decoding visions, tracking soul whispers, or just letting the ink remember what your heart already knows.)*

PART 3. HEAL

TAKING FLIGHT

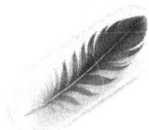

It's not that I have power, but when I pray, I pray with the right motivation. Motivation is the key. If you have the right motivation, then a lot of positive things can happen that are not explained.

—Grandmother Tsering Dolma Gyaltong (Tibet)

I was formally initiated into shamanism through the Q'ero shaman lineage by Dr. Peter Bonaker, an energy medicine practitioner I met through The Four Winds Society. My experiences working alongside him—as a friend, teacher, and mentor—inspired me to become a Certified End of Life Doula.[29] Through Peter, I learned how to hold sacred space for those in transition, guiding them not only through the physical experience of death, but also through the emotional and spiritual journey of moving from one dimension to the next. It was through his teachings that I came to understand the profound role of a shaman in creating a safe environment for inner work, allowing clients to meet their fears, release old wounds, and open to deeper healing.

One of the most transformative concepts I learned from Peter was the view of time in shamanism. In Western cultures, we often see time as linear—a series of events, with past, present, and future in a straight line. However, in shamanic healing, time is circular.[30] This cyclical view of time enables us to have a more expansive perspective, where our past, present, and future interconnect, are fluid, and continuously influence each other.

This concept became especially meaningful to me during my training, where Peter shared the symbolism of the **Circled Cross**.

The Circled Cross, two crisscrossed lines within a circle, is a universal symbol of infinite time and an ancient symbol of the shaman's universe. Also known as **the circular cross**, it is found in lands as far removed as the Celts of the British Isles and the Mapuche of Chile, South America. The lines represent the four directions moving out into infinity, and the center point from which the shaman moves. Each direction is associated with a purpose and a life epoch. In the Q'ero tradition, the South represents our past. The West represents the ability to travel beyond death. The North represents our ancestors, and the East represents our connection with *Spirit* and our future.

For many centuries, people relied on the healing gifts that their medicine people or village shamans offered. A shaman recognizes that any physical pain and emotional distress can originate back in time, through time and space, either through ancestral DNA or from injuries suffered in previous incarnations. A shaman learns to travel through time and space and can influence an outcome and remove the origin of a trauma as he or she travels in circular time.

Through my experiences with Peter, I learned that a shaman's role is not just to provide healing, but also to become a bridge between time and dimensions, guiding clients through their inner journeys. It is through the deep connections we build as shamans that we can hold sacred space for others, helping them confront unresolved traumas from the past or fears about their future. Whether through energetic healing, guidance, or simply being present, the shaman's journey through time opens the door to transformation.

The work of healing is deeply relational. Just like a flight to a different time zone, our souls yearn for deep connection with others—a connection that transcends time and space. By understanding the struggles and wounds that people face—whether rooted in the past, carried from previous lives, or shaped by ancestral trauma—we can identify ways to support their inner healing.

Success on this journey depends on the strength of the connection. By addressing both past and present challenges, a shaman can help clients open to healthier relationships with themselves and others, ultimately creating a brighter future. The connection we offer as healers is not just about applying techniques, but about recognizing the weight of what others bear. Understanding the root of their struggles allows us to be more effective in facilitating healing and guiding them on their path. Through this understanding, we empower others to release old wounds and make space for unconditional love—first for themselves, and then for others.

The teachings of Dr. Peter Bonaker, along with the wisdom of the Q'ero, illuminated for me the importance of love, connection, and the continuous flow of time. Healing is not just about mending what is broken—it's about remembering our interconnectedness and realizing that every moment, every connection, and every experience holds healing potential. Through this deep, sacred understanding, we can step into a more expansive role in the lives of others, allowing their healing to become part of our own. This shared journey fosters a kind of healing that transcends time, making the present moment one of infinite possibilities for growth, love, and transformation.

STORY FROM THE HEALING TABLE: REWRITING THE MIND-BODY CONVERSATION

The joys of life can be easily overridden by negative stress stemming from self-imposed restrictions that should improve outcomes, yet often do the opposite. These choices can lead to guilt and shame. A person might proclaim they're on a diet, sit down to dinner, stop themselves from reaching for another piece of bread, then take it anyway. When they do, they may eat it with a sense of wrongdoing. Someone might order a glass of wine and immediately judge it as a vice instead of seeing it as a portal to appreciation. There can be anxiety that every indulgence is damaging or shortening life. For some, pleasure feels like something to be sacrificed to escape suffering. In those cases, shame and guilt can quietly stow away in the body.

The pain-body concept is central in Energy Medicine, referring to an accumulation of energetic blockages springing from emotional pain. It's like an internal demonic force that lives inside the healed body, the low vibes overtaking the high vibes. Author Eckhart Tolle describes the pain-body in his bestselling book, A New Earth, as an "energy field of old but still very much alive emotion that lives in almost every human being."[31] It is conditional, in the same way we think love demands something from us. It influences our thoughts, feelings, and behaviors.

I stayed in an emotionally turbulent, loveless marriage out of duty, hoping that my efforts would make her love me. Our relationship to consumption, body image, and getting older is no different. Our decisions either take up or free up space in our bodies' connective tissues. How do we know that the human body can heal itself?

> The human energy system comprises physical, emotional, mental, and spiritual dimensions. Within this framework, the **pain body** is considered an energetic residue of past emotional traumas, unresolved conflicts, and suppressed negative experiences. It is considered an energetic counterpart to physical pain, manifesting in various forms and affecting different aspects of health.

Healing cannot be dependent only on doctors or a scientific cure. It springs from your inner guidance system that greets the fear-based world, knowing anything is possible. By seeing everything we take in and give back as medicine, we can open space to live a long and healthy life.

Michele first came to me, referring to chronic migraines and severe menstrual cramps. She told me that even when she didn't have a headache, she felt a constant pressure in her temples that was negatively impacting her quality of life. Moody and miserable, she told me that to get through the day, she had to pretend past her pain so it wouldn't be detectable at work. After searching for over a year, she was unable to find a cure.

Research has shown that headaches are associated with loss of control.[32] People who focus on control eventually lose the battle and burn out because not all problems can be solved with intellect. Going to illogical spaces can feel off-limits for those with controlling tendencies. The longer they take to develop ways to cope with the unknown, the longer they forgo treatment for what ails them.

Emotions and bodily pain are interconnected.[33] When we experience emotional distress, such as anxiety, sadness, or stress, it can manifest as physical pain. This connection is because of the brain's role in processing emotional and physical pain, often through shared neural pathways.

Emotional pain can trigger the release of stress hormones like cortisol, which may lead to inflammation or muscle tension, resulting in physical discomfort. Negative emotional states can exacerbate or trigger chronic pain conditions, creating a feedback loop where pain and emotions feed into each other.

Phantom pain is a phenomenon where individuals who have lost a limb continue to feel sensations, including pain, in the area where the limb used to be. This pain is real and can be quite debilitating, even though the limb is no longer physically present. Phantom pain occurs because the brain's neural map of the body remains intact, even after the loss of a limb. The brain continues signaling to the missing limb, leading to the sensation of pain. You can also think of it like the concept of generational patterning referenced in Part 1. Before we know it, we are filled with cling-ons that become attached to our DNA.

This concept extends beyond the physical into the emotional and psychological realms. As the brain struggles to adjust to the loss of a limb, it also grapples with emotional losses or disappointments. The attachment to what was lost—whether a relationship, a dream, or a loved one—can create a form of "phantom pain" in the psyche, where the person continues to feel the emotional pain associated with the loss.

Energy Medicine is based on the idea that the body and mind are composed of energy fields that can be influenced to promote healing. In working with emotional pain, Energy Medicine addresses subtle vibrational imbalances that arise from emotional attachments and disappointments. These imbalances can manifest as physical pain, emotional distress, or a sense of being "stuck" in the past.

The process of detaching from these emotional attachments is analogous to the brain's need to rewire itself after the loss of a limb. As the brain eventually learns to stop sending pain signals to the missing limb, emotional detachment involves releasing the energy associated with the loss, allowing the person to move forward.

Detaching from emotional pain is a gradual process that involves recognizing and releasing the attachment to the source of pain. This can be achieved through various methods, including mindfulness, exploring different types of psychotherapy, meditation, and energy healing practices such as Reiki or acupuncture. These practices help to rebalance the body's energy and reduce the emotional "phantom pain" that lingers after a loss. By addressing and releasing these attachments, individuals can ease emotional and physical pain, leading to a greater sense of peace and well-being.

Michele told me on her first visit to my healing table that she felt the pressure release in her head for the first time as far back as she could remember. Having grown up in an abusive household, the trauma she experienced with the mood swings of her father erupting into complete chaos, she believed, had caused her to cope by exerting control.

Our work together helped her understand that her emotions were being stored in her body. After I'd cleared the energetic imprint stuck in her auric field around her head, she was able to begin meditating regularly, creating new boundaries in her relationships, and forming healthy habits related to nutrition and movement that helped her clear her energy every morning. After releasing the trapped emotions that had been stored in her body since childhood, Michele began making new decisions about how she was living her life. Eventually, like many healing arts professionals and I, she embarked on a new professional pathway to become an Energy Medicine practitioner.

The relationship between emotions and bodily pain is complex and multifaceted. Phantom pain illustrates how the brain holds onto pain signals even after a physical loss, and this concept can be extended to emotional pain as well. Energy Medicine offers tools to help release these attachments, facilitating healing and reducing pain in the body and mind. Only when the pain subsides, or even better, when it goes away, do we create space for the long and healthy life we seek to live.

7

EMBODYING AUTHENTICITY: SUSTAINING HEALTH IN A TOXIC WORLD

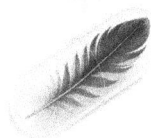

T he most reassuring thing about healing is that it's the natural mode of operation of the body. When one of our cells dies, another one is born. It's a chance to begin again, to regenerate, given to us in the biological makeup of our human hood. Our skin cells are replaced every few weeks. If you donate your liver, up to two-thirds of it will be given to the recipient. Within only six to eight weeks, it will grow back to its original size. On an even larger scale, the entirety of our cellular makeup is renewed every seven to ten years. Why is it that more people than ever are suffering from chronic and autoimmune diseases, struggling to find a cure or even a diagnosis?

Disease is characterized as "any harmful deviation from the normal structural or functional state of an organism. It is generally associated with certain signs and symptoms differing in nature from physical injury."[34]

To comprehend how dis-ease impacts our everyday lives, we have to understand our "normal," or what I would say is our natural or authentic state of being. This leads to aligning our actions with what we say we want. When we think, consume, and act in a direct line, this dis-ease subsides. A large part of this is nourishment.

We all want access to healthy, local, organic produce. Yet supermarkets are filled with processed foods and ingredients, which you need to decipher through struggling to read the small print on the back label before knowing whether you should eat them. Factory farming and fast food have wreaked havoc on our culture, and pesticide pollution is at an all-time high. Don't get me wrong, this isn't a full-blown assault against farmers or a political statement. It's a realization stemming from a human being trying to live a long and healthy life that many factors play against this. When we combine the difficulty of finding healthy options with the fear-based world that is ever-present through our smartphones, it's easy to see how we are constantly feeling like we are running from a tiger. There's doom and gloom everywhere, and getting discouraged or sidetracked is easier than ever.

The good news is that we are becoming more informed and aware of the science behind stress and its impact on our lives, both negative and positive. Because we have the knowledge and desire to be healthy, there's no better time to mend our relationship with the bad information we eat, drink, and read that is present in our daily lives. Healing happens on the cellular level. Have our environment, circumstances, and new cultural norms, like online scrolling, temporarily disfigured our cellular makeup? When we sit across from our friend at dinner, who is also scrolling, is the social disconnection we experience working against our bodies' natural abilities to heal? In my experience, it was. I invite you to answer this question for yourself.

There is no linear path to healing. At first, it is the line of chaos on the graph, with jagged edges jutting up and plummeting down. This is normal when you have left yourself behind or ruminated on past hurts inflicted on you, like I did.

Developing awareness that allows access to intuition so you can understand where the existential guideposts are asking you to go, the line softens into a rolling hill. Eventually, it develops into an EKG of a healthy heart. Learning what we are genuinely made of and how to employ our authentic selves leads us to understand the source from which unconditional love is conceived. We don't only make different choices when we heal on this energetic basis. We take spirited action and see what life offers us and what we choose to receive as medicine.

The Truth in the Mirror

Sold on the premise of healing others through my private practice, little did I know the important role my home would play in my healing from cancer. It became so much more than I imagined. My adult treehouse was surrounded by towering tulip poplars and oak trees, with a little creek running through the property line. Deer and foxes were visible from the kitchen window. After moving in, I renovated and redesigned the rooms, giving me a sense of satisfaction and creating a space that invited me to burn sage and play the drums again. Shortly after I moved in, I realized it was the perfect time to recreate the positive feelings from childhood that I had on those Sunday mornings with my family.

My strategy was to double down on my healing activities outside the office, to counter the negative impact on me. Sundays became a huge part of that. I would work all week, and on the seventh day, wake up without an alarm, light candles, turn on classical music, and press the button on my European espresso machine before turning on CBS News Sunday Morning. Silencing my phone and creating a work-free zone, the simplicity and the quiet were the highlights of my week.

As my healing work expanded and contributed to a sense of self I had never found through my "day job," the corporate world was more demoralizing and stressful than ever. The tension I felt reverberated beyond the 9–5 workday. It was difficult to feel like my energy was split between two worlds. Even though I was pain-free, the contradiction between my two worlds was like Dr. Jekyll and Mr. Hyde. In many ways, I was still hiding. While I kept the title of Reiki Master on my public platforms, I was not promoting my work. Very few people, outside of the clients who came to my healing practice, understood the scope of my work. It wasn't only about the work I was doing. It was about the life I was carving out for myself.

In solitude in the treehouse, I tapped into my artistic side, and a man who creates vision board collages and spins pottery emerged. When I went to work, there was no sign of the person I was with at home. I knew that exposing all of who I am in corporate America would threaten my reputation and further risk being taken seriously. Going to work was a logical space with expectations of men in leadership that I always had a hard time fulfilling. I kept convincing myself it was worth hanging on to corporate America, mainly for financial security.

One particular Sunday morning, as I watched the spring showers rain down through a large window from the living room, feeling like one of those contemplative characters in the movies, I noticed a familiar sensation in the back of my throat. The same sensation I had on my first visit to the doctor to inspect the lump behind my uvula.

I swallowed a few more times and feverishly rose from the couch. Has it returned? I hoped it was all in my head. Irritated, I walked toward the bathroom, throwing out expletives. How stupid was I to think I was safe to be content so soon after I beat this thing? Why did I get sick every time I felt well? This lump was not supposed to come back. No, this fucking lump was not supposed to come back. It deserves to be addressed as a curse.

Turning on the light above the sink, it wasn't bright enough. I scrambled back to the kitchen, rushing past the burning candles I had lit an hour before when I started my awesomely predictable, main-character Sunday morning routine. I quickly grabbed a butter knife from the silverware drawer and my iPhone from the charging station. Walking the three-foot plank back to the bathroom, I continued to swear over Yo-Yo Ma's hopeful rendition of "Bach's Cello Suite No. 1 in G Major" playing in the background.

Posturing myself against the front of the sink, I turned on the flashlight on my phone. Placing the butter knife on my tongue like one of those wooden sticks doctors use before they have you say, "Ahhh," I moved my head around to find the perfect position to see the back of my throat through the mirror. My mouth was wide open, and my fingers were tensely wrapped around the butter knife.

Yep, there it was again—a round growth the size of a marble jutting out from the red soft tissue in the back of my throat behind my uvula (that teardrop-shaped, dangling thing). It wasn't strep. It wasn't a regrown tonsil. That lump was the same one that was cancerous.

Letting the knife drop to the floor in defeat, walking back to the living room, I considered that this thing had come back to take my life. My parents rushed me to the hospital at three years old, barely breathing. The glass in my face when the drunk driver hit our car, and the motorcycle accident, all paled compared to the thought of going through cancer again.

When was it going to stop?

The chemo, the trips to Germany, being replaced and reassigned to a lackluster project at work, and the threat of losing my life were not things I wanted to face again. The lump was back, threatening everything I had done to heal. I felt anger boiling up inside of me. I knew I had to allow myself to move through it. If I accepted it, I wouldn't get stuck in the feeling, and I trusted I would eventually find clarity. I sat with my rage for the rest of the day. The left side of my brain was predicting my death, watching my kids look at me in a casket, the guy who failed them, the man who failed himself, too. As I calmed down, I heard my inner voice. It assured and comforted me with Grandmother Rita's words; my hands could heal. My health was in my hands.

Too often, we dismiss low-vibrational emotions, but I have learned that they are useful. In my anger, I found the questions that would lead me to answers that would, as I had projected a year earlier, crumble my reality.

What if this lump was calling me to the next level of my healing?

What if it was saving my life?

Why was I spending half of my waking life in a career that was off-purpose?

I knew that the notion that life was happening to me was more bad information. Everything happened for me. I believed this with every cell in my body.

I had to mend my physical body to open myself up to heal the emotional, mental, and spiritual dimensions of my health. Or was it that I had to mend the emotional and mental wounds to open up to physical healing? The energy was all connected. It didn't matter which came first. Quitting my job would heal me in all dimensions. If I stayed, the stress would block me from living a life at full capacity. Having been granted the opportunity to live repeatedly, I couldn't take that for granted.

"Feel the anger and transcend," I told myself.

Words That Saved Me

I had allowed my bosses to reassign me from a project I had created, without standing up for myself, taking it like a man who didn't value himself, and repeatedly becoming sick. In my earlier years, I was part of a company culture where everyone on the team said their blood ran the logo's color. I considered that to be crazier than any of my spiritual explorations.

You might expect me to tell you I marched into work the next morning and turned in my notice. That didn't happen. I stayed for nearly two more years, continuing to conjure different answers to those questions I had asked in anger. While I changed many areas of my life, the thought of leaving my job was one I had to weigh more heavily. I could look back and scold myself for not creating an exit strategy sooner, but I've learned that sometimes, action is only sparked by gale-force winds. Just like in nature, energy often rushes from high-pressure systems into low-pressure ones—powerfully and without hesitation.

I decided to make it impossible for this lump to survive, solve the riddle, and find the root cause of what it was trying to show me. I could only do that if I never returned to the office again. As I continued digging, I returned to the power of words. "I love myself. I accept myself. I love you. I love you. I love you. I love you." The words of affirmation I had used in the past saw me through some of the worst times in my life. To get that lump out of my throat, I would once again use language to heal.

One psychic I worked with kept pointing out that "Cancer is not in your future." I explained to her that because colon cancer had run in my family, my mother always reminded us to make sure we went in for regular checkups and cancer screenings.

"The Universe doesn't understand the word no or not," she said. She continued to point out that the law of attraction depends only on words, defining what you want to have happen. By including the word cancer, I was attracting it. I created a new affirmation.

"I live a long and healthy life. I am healthy." I said this out loud relentlessly for ten days. On the 11th day, the lump disappeared. I confirmed it was gone using the same butter knife-to-tongue method I used that rainy Sunday morning. When I saw my oncologist, she confirmed it was gone, too.

A series of fortunate events culminated in my eventual resignation from my job. When I left the company, I knew it was for good, and traded in the position in the C-Suite for a role over the healing table.

After my pending departure became public, a close friend congratulated me. "Go shine[IP]," she said. There wasn't a good-bye party or a slew of messages of gratitude exchanged on my last day in corporate America. I moved through a lot of grief and sadness, knowing my departure was not only the death of the role I played at work. My ego was slain, and it was the best thing that ever happened to me. I took her words with me and left the rest behind.

Looking back, going to work filled my body with environmental toxins. I pride myself on being an empathetic leader who recognizes others' strengths. Treating people with kindness was a weakness. I did not fit into the business landscape of the organizations I worked for. Even though I wasn't sure what would come from my time in corporate America, I knew it was fuel to eventually build something useful out of the rubble. The next company I would create would be mine, and the culture would not punish team members for being sick.

My work in product development translated into a helpful lesson for how I would approach my life. When I built software, I was trained to direct the development based on what the company wanted the "users" of the product to think, say, and do. It was time to take the knowledge I gained and apply it to my life. What do I think, feel, do, and say about my life? The lessons I learned by using affirmative language began showing up again. This time, I could begin translating that work into rewriting the entirety of my life story by using affirmative language again intentionally.

Leaving the pain-body I continuously revisited throughout my life meant it could now be healed of chronic dis-ease. Not only was my healing practice expanding, but my sensibilities and sensitivities made me a father whose adult children felt comfortable confiding in me about the struggles they were facing. I could be there for them in a way I never had before. The richness of my creativity called in friends who enjoyed coming to my home to eat a meal I cooked for them with love. They thought I was great at chopping onions.

My healed body proudly awaited me in this new world I was designing.

"You get to live this long and healthy life," I told myself.

A new question arose.

Now, what more are you going to make of it?

READER REFLECTION: ALIGNING YOUR LIFE WITH AUTHENTICITY

What areas of your life or circumstances are leaving you feeling unfulfilled, beat up, powerless, or victimized right now?

What lessons might these areas of your life or circumstances be trying to teach you?

How is life happening for you, as opposed to happening to you?

How can what's happening for you align with the way you are living your life with your authentic self?

ACTIONABLE INSIGHTS TO HEAL ACROSS FOUR DIMENSIONS OF HEALTH

Emotional

Embracing the highs and lows of your emotional journey, you can use anger and frustration as catalysts to uncover deeper truths and align your life with your authentic self.

Mental

Shifting your mindset by using positive affirmations and reframing your internal dialogue allows your thoughts to guide you toward healing and growth.

Physical

Paying attention to your body's signals and making conscious decisions to nurture it through both traditional and alternative approaches fosters long-term health and vitality.

Spiritual

Trusting in existential guideposts and spiritual practices like affirmations and energy healing supports your journey toward alignment and purpose.

SPIRITED ACT OF AUTHENTICITY: POSITIVE AFFIRMATIONS

When I was going through my healing phase after my auto-immune diagnosis, a good friend of mine suggested reading Louise Hay's book, *You Can Heal Your Body*.[35] I hadn't heard of her then, and was intrigued by the simplicity of her findings. I encourage you to read some of her books, as Louise has had an equally interesting life story. Her findings that you can heal yourself with positive affirmations are profound, yet so simple in their application. I've been saying throughout this book that self-love is one of the most important aspects of our healing journey.

My second learning was to be mindful of our thoughts, as some might manifest themselves unintentionally. There is a fascinating new finding that epigenetics is the cause of what, in earlier years, were believed to be family diseases. Think about what we're told by the medical community: "Oh, your dad died of colon cancer, so you should get regular colonoscopies, as you are at a higher risk of getting it too." That's what happened to me, and subsequently, I told myself regularly: "Cancer isn't in my future." I've desired a cancer-free life, but I now believe that having the "C" word in my vocabulary daily multiple times might have caused my cancer, not genetics or inherited family DNA.

When my lump returned, I started to change my manifestation from "Cancer isn't in my future" to "I live a long and healthy life, I am healthy." The same desired outcome, but different phrasing. And I healed myself within *ten days*. It's a different vibe, right? That's where the topic of epigenetics comes in. Could it be that by changing our narrative from a low-vibe, fear-based thought pattern to a high-vibe, positive affirmation, we can heal ourselves naturally? Give it a try. You might be surprised by how much your mind can help you stay healthy.

Here are some of my favorite affirmations that I use to this day.

> *I love myself, I love myself, I love myself.*
> *I approve of myself, I approve of myself, I approve of myself.*
> *I live a long and healthy life. I am healthy.*
> *All of life comes to me with ease, joy, and glory.*

Sacred Scribbles *(Use these pages as a portal for decoding visions, tracking soul whispers, or just letting the ink remember what your heart already knows.)*

8

THE LIFE SPIRAL: MAKING
PEACE WITH TRANSITIONS

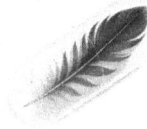

When a child is born, everyone rallies. We host baby showers and christenings. Photos are continuously taken in admiration of watching our children develop. Yet, there are rarely celebrations regarding the end of this life. As we age, we remark on the deterioration of our bodies, the wrinkles, and the creaky joints. We anticipate disease because we are told we are genetically vulnerable, or the statistics are against us.

Knowing that life as we know it will end for all of us, there is a big void and gap in our society. The more we listen and watch, the more we absorb the outside world as a fact of life. We speak of the past as the culmination of the joy we will never experience again. For some, death means the end of the story; for others, like me, it's a precursor to what's next. No matter what you believe, could it be that, anticipating death, we dismiss the incredible fact that we are still alive and have more to experience?

If you are tempted to turn away from this chapter out of discomfort with talking about the end of life as we know it, I invite you to stay and move through the beliefs you've formed.

You might decide those beliefs aren't yours to hold anymore. The prospect that you will make peace with death by reading a few pages of a book, I realize, is highly unlikely. Living life more joyfully because of the exploration of the end of it, I hope, will begin to unfold in your mind, body, and soul.

You have come this far. There's more clearing to do and more false conditioning to rise above. The deeper you go, the higher your life extends. Consider the length of your long and healthy life, the distance between you and outer space. While many of us want to maximize our time here on earth, I ask you to consider that energy is the fuel to help you go the vertical distance. Ultimately, the higher we travel, the more our lives form around our purpose.

INTO THE SPIRITUAL REALM

My brother, Valentin, actively manifests his long and healthy lifespan of 120 years. Me? I just want to live it up.

My decisions until I was in my late forties were all based on fear of the past. The career that made me sick, the love that wasn't unconditional, and the lack of care I gave to my physical and emotional health were all based on the thinking that I had to achieve certain levels of material success before I died. Realizing this, I was not living every day. I was dying, dying to be seen instead of living on purpose.

So, how do we rid our lives of the slow erosion of meaning? We undergo a cellular death so we can transform.

A few years after attending the Grow a New Body Retreat, where I faced my mortality, I read Alberto Villoldo's book, *Shaman, Healer, Sage*. I had begun my shamanic training, and I knew that I had to connect with death and dying through the spiritual realm to be equipped to fully access the breadth of the teachings I was being entrusted to translate into the Western world. I was reminded of my family's conversations on Sunday mornings around the table. I recall my mom reading a quote from Elisabeth Kübler-Ross aloud: "It is not the end of the physical body that should worry us. Rather, our concern must be to live while we're alive—to release our inner selves from the spiritual death that comes with living behind a façade designed to conform to external definitions of who and what we are."

The past sure has a way of suddenly making a lot of sense.

In his book, Villoldo describes the process of the death spiral, a call to construct a pathway to transitioning beyond this reality while we are still alive.[36] The intricacies of what I read sent me down a rabbit hole. When I came up for air, it was clear I wanted to help souls pass into the spiritual realm after their earthly death. There was more that I wanted to offer. I knew that families needed guidance to see them through the process of grief that begins well before their loved one takes their last breath.

After asking myself what more I could do with my long and healthy life, I decided to become a Certified End-of-Life Doula through Doulagivers Institute™, founded by Suzanne O'Brien.[37] A "Death Doula," similar to a Birth Doula, is a conduit between a patient's medical care team and their family. Doulas work with people who have been given a terminal diagnosis.

One of the first times I went to the bedside, it was next to the father of a friend of mine. When I arrived, his hands were clenched tightly around the bed railings. Even as he drifted in and out of sleep under the influence of morphine, he held on.

Witnessing the signs of distress, I asked him for permission. "May I touch you? I am here to help you relax. Are you open to receiving my help?" I spoke softly.

He moved his head up and down ever so slightly in confirmation. As I lit a bundle of white sage, and the smoke formed around his body, he opened his eyes, looked at me, and said with a smirk, "1963, dude."

While I laughed in the moment, I also understood it marked the early stages of his dying—drawing him back through memory as he slowly released his hold on life. He was clearing the time that was stored in his body.

One of the ancient practices I've learned in my shamanic training is removing stored and stuck energies from people's bodies. It's like a magnetic cord that pulls all of the trauma, regrets, and perceived sins from a patient's auric field. Starting with the root chakra, moving through the sacral chakra before finishing at the crown, he revealed parts of his life in subtle sounds and more ambiguous (and sometimes humorous) one-liners that indicated he was letting go of experiences that hid in the caverns of his body. To keep what was happening private and sacred, I will refrain from specifics, but imagine everything you have hidden for fear of the judgment of the outside world exiting your body. What an incredible relief.

Before my mother passed, a love story she had tucked away before she married my father came to the surface. There was nothing shameful about it, but out of respect for my dad, the pictures of the memories she had with a man she loved before him were destroyed after they met. Memories far exceed the lifespan of a Polaroid. The photo albums left in the boxes in the attic, when opened up through the surgical removal of energetic imprints, allow us to let go in compassionate remembrance of our time here.

As my work with my friend's father ended, I recalled that his family had told me he didn't like his feet to be touched. When I finished the chakra clearing, I reconnected with him, touching his feet. He was not bothered in the least. His body was entirely at peace. A sudden vibrational current sent waves of overwhelmingly positive energy through my hands. It was like a frequency to my favorite classic rock station, 103.7 FM. He served as an antenna, communicating unconditional love through a tower that reached an elevation the eye could not see.

This feeling of absolute peace, joy, and love is often described by patients who have had near-death experiences.

For a moment, I forgot about the fear-based world myself. In the process of healing him and helping him pass, he gave me the greatest gift ever: having access to this divine love. No longer holding onto the side of the bed, he peacefully passed two days later. His widow called me the following day to tell me that the pillow she had taken from his bed was emitting the colors of the rainbow in the dark of night. In the days following, she would later share that the colors faded.

After my work with my friend's father, my desire to help people transition grew. I set out to make sure that people departing the earth would be given the chance to alleviate their pain, loosen their grip, and find relief from the low-vibrational energetic footprint that was asking them to hold on to dear life. Too many of us are living with emotional gunk and sludge that, when processed, can make the dying process more comfortable and the journey peaceful and safe. In the work that I do as a Death Doula, I wonder what would happen if more people became comfortable with death, as soon as we are given life, to make being alive feel more peaceful and safe.

I Can Heal Myself

What if we choose to die an emotional death every day, releasing the toxic thought patterns that burden us with rampant thoughts of moments we regret, the "shoulds," and the "what ifs?" We can regenerate and repair our cellular structure by choosing new thoughts that we speak in affirmative words.

If we look back, wishing life were different, we are digging ourselves a shallow grave. If we look back so we can understand ourselves on a deeper level and make something great out of every mistake, mishap, or tragedy, we are in a state of purpose. Our death is rooted, upholding the legacy of our lives. Every human desires to feel healthy, yet many miss the opportunity to feel like it. We think it's too late or our time has passed, but time only exists right here, right now.

We wonder why we are alive. The answer lies in the energetic movement of emotions. By making sense of our past, we can find purpose at any age, even moments before we die. I hope to help you do this now. Wherever you are in life, it is never too late. We think we live every day, but when false conditioning and bad information are compounding in our bodies, we merely exist, risking becoming figments of our past instead of statements of our purpose.

What if we could see death as a positive part of life? An extension of the world we are living in now. Whether you believe in an afterlife or not, you will leave something behind from your time here: a memory, a company, a family.

Has the desire to become healthy been blocked by the fear-based world, like it was for me? Expectations placed on us by our parents that we cannot fulfill, low body image from the bullies or societal standards that greet us in the media, unsustainable quick-fix diet programs, or financially unattainable means of being healthy, remove us from our power.

Purpose places us in the most important state of our existence because through it, we understand who we are and why we are here. Being in a state of purpose is not defined by what you do, but rather a feeling you generate by transforming your emotional state from a low vibration to higher-toned thoughts and actions. A state of purpose invites trust, unconditional love, and health into your life because it is not a demand. It is a magnetic pull to your heart.

My own journey with a mysterious illness taught me how many layers healing can have. When I relied solely on steroids for a few months, they'd give me temporary relief—I'd feel like I could dance on tables—but when they wore off, the pain often felt worse than before. This was my experience with surface-level solutions. I want to be clear: if you take prescription medicine, I'm not suggesting you stop. What I discovered for myself was that exploring energetic and epigenetic factors opened up new dimensions of healing I hadn't considered before. If you're curious about looking deeper into your own health journey, you might discover, as I did, entirely new ways of experiencing wellness.

The truth about healing is that you can go as fast or as slowly as you please. You might even enjoy it if you are in a state of purpose. The art I create heals me. Not every spirited act of healing is a deep dive into our past lives. Blissfully engaging with our present is equally beneficial. Once you begin seeing your life for what it is, when you show up as your full-throttle self, full of opportunities disguised as misfortunes, everything changes for the better. Life begins to work for you when you see that the evidence supports that it always has.

When I say I could heal myself, and you can too, I mean it wholeheartedly. When we proclaim, "I can heal myself," there is power. When we wait for the answers and lean into only the opinions, statistics, and recommendations of others, we neglect the full range of possibilities out there to explore that can improve our lives.

I would argue that the majority of people feel physically imbalanced or in pain because they can't see what they can't see. Emotions are visible only in reactions and responses that are too often harshly judged by the world. A powerful way to understand emotions is to feel them through the body, to be with them quietly, and allow them to be heard and understood. Your intuition speaks through your physicality. Spirit, the Universe, God, energy…whatever you want to call it, is waiting to communicate with you.

"So what if people think you are nuts?" More supportive words gifted to me by the friend who had told me to "Go Shine" ricocheted back to me as if they were now mine. She responded to my admission that there was still a little voice from the fear-based world inside my head. I told her that a small part of me was mulling over the potential judgment of my spiritual explorations from the fear-based world around me. She reminded me that one of the existential guideposts of my life was the lengthy amount of time I had spent in the travel industry. "Now you are issuing the last boarding pass for people passing on to the other side," she said.

Elated by the metaphor, I recalled how much I enjoyed plane travel but decided to turn it up a notch. It was time to go to space.

READER REFLECTION: LIVING IT UP HERE ON EARTH

If you could go back in time, what memories would you most enjoy living over again?

What regrets do you have in your life? Is there anyone that you need to forgive? Is there anyone that you need forgiveness from? Is there anyone that you need to tell that you love them?

How can you make peace with your regrets?

How can you create more memories that give you the feeling of your most enjoyable moments?

ACTIONABLE INSIGHTS TO HEAL ACROSS FOUR DIMENSIONS OF HEALTH

Emotional

By releasing toxic thought patterns and embracing your present reality, you open up the possibility for healing and personal transformation, leading to greater emotional balance.

Mental

Shifting your perspective by viewing life's challenges as opportunities for growth helps you mentally align with your purpose and break free from limiting beliefs.

Physical

Understanding that your body is a reflection of your emotional and mental health, and by mending the pain within, you can restore physical vitality and well-being.

Spiritual

Exploring the deeper meanings of life, including death, as a way to reconnect with your true purpose and spirit, allows you to live more openly and peacefully.

SPIRITED ACT OF AUTHENTICITY: CHANGE YOUR NARRATIVE—FROM HIGH VIBE DAY TO HIGH VIBE LIFE

Have you ever intentionally thought about the personal stories you've been telling yourself about your life? Most of us come with a good amount of baggage and trauma. Whether you've grown up with divorced parents, had an abusive partner, or were hit with an illness or accident, we all carry the stories of pain and suffering with us. In my client work, I often observe someone telling me something like, "I am unable to do 'Y' until 'X' has resolved itself."

We seem to be prisoners of our own stories, believing that change must come from outside us or that an event must occur before we can step into our power and heal. This is another "lie" that the fear-based world has us believe. If you wait for situations, seasons, or other people to change to give yourself permission to take action, you might get stuck. This is common in many facets of our healing and growth. An example might be waiting to shed the five pounds until the holidays are over. Then, when the holidays are over, you have to wait until after your kid's birthday, and after that, there is another event or thing that has to happen.

Our dreams die as we wait for the world around us to somehow make it easier or grant us the perfect moment. Waiting without taking action can lead to a paralyzing and powerless feeling. I am offering up another narrative, one that is full of hope and healing, but even more than that, is action-based. Once we change our narrative and story, we have the foundation for manifesting the life we're meant to live. However, it is more than a thought or word. It is how the thoughts and words are constructed that inspires us to act in alignment with the way the narratives are formed.

I believe we shape our human existence through the dialogue we have with ourselves, with others, and with the world around us—including a higher universal power. Reframing what we speak and the energetic vibration we put out into the world manifests our destiny. It begins with speaking on behalf of the long and healthy lives we want to live, leads to internalizing a new belief system based on unconditional self-love, and culminates in the meaning and purpose we find in our existence. Telling new and inspiring stories removes the shackles of the past and releases the blame we place on others, allowing us to launch our rocket into space. But first, we must understand the stories we tell ourselves.

I invite you to grab a journal, a cup of tea, and something to write with and make yourself comfortable in front of your altar, if you have created one, or a quiet space where you feel most comfortable.

- Light a candle and ponder the following thoughts.
    - What happened to me?
    - Who is responsible?
    - How did it change my life?
    - How has it influenced my behavior?

    Keep asking similar questions and writing the answers out. Please don't judge yourself. Inquiry isn't about finding answers to place blame; it's about getting to the core of your current beliefs.

Once you feel the process is complete, please give yourself time before the next step. The amount of time is up to you. You may want to go for a walk to clear your mind, get a massage, or go to the spa if you need it. Right now is a time to just "be" in the present moment and observe your feelings about what you wrote down. When you feel ready to revisit this, I encourage you to look at what you wrote with compassion for yourself and the people you wrote about.

- The final step of this process is to see what's possible and write about the possibilities without feeling like something has to change first. This may sound a little foreign at first, but with a little practice, you will start to change your narrative.

- o Reflect on what you wrote down. Circle all words that you believe carry a low vibration. List them on the left-hand side of a separate sheet of paper.

- o Next, place a box around all of the high-vibrational words you wrote down, and list those on the right-hand side of the separate sheet of paper alongside the low-vibrational words.

- o How many low-vibrational words versus high-vibrational words did you use? Use this for awareness.

- Write down the high-vibrational opposite or antonym for all low-vibrational words. Some examples might be "can't" to "can" or "didn't" to "do" or "ugly" to "beautiful" or "failure" to "success." Again, use this to increase awareness of how to reframe words.

- Next, complete the following by using only high-vibrational words.

Because _____ happened to me, I learned _____, and now I can use that learning to _____.

An example of mine would be, "Because I got cancer, I learned so much about healthcare and healing, and now I can use that learning to help other people heal."

The purpose of this exercise is to dream big. To imagine what your life could look like if you're no longer held back by limiting beliefs. It's about not making excuses and avoiding speaking of things that seem impossible or you believe will never work.

Think of humankind designing a rocket. It all started with a dream to be on the moon. Had these inventors not had a conviction that they could do it, even though it seemed impossible, they would have never started to build the rocket. The same is true for you: Imagine a life of limitless achievement and abundance. Write it out, and use the vision board exercise in Chapter 9 to properly manifest. It's time to instill a new belief system. One that tells you that anything is possible.

Sacred Scribbles *(Use these pages as a portal for decoding visions, tracking soul whispers, or just letting the ink remember what your heart already knows.)*

9

FAITH IN THE UNSEEN: LIVING ONWARD AND UPWARD

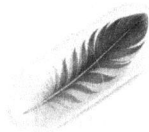

Before I could live authentically, I had to learn to listen to my intuition and pay attention to the existential guideposts.

Before being loved unconditionally, I had to create high-vibrational response systems that established trust in my relationships.

Before I could heal, I had to take spirited actions on purpose.

Before I could transcend the fear-based world, I had to create wide-open spaces for the natural forces I could not see.

When I was born, I met the fear-based world.

Growing up, I learned to adopt it as my living truth.

It told me to strive for outer success and belonging.

I created a list of wants and desires that were not mine.

I got a lot of what I wanted, but I became confused by why I continued to feel unfulfilled.

I suffered and kept wondering why my life was being threatened.

And then, somewhere between living and dying, I discovered that everything I want is in the palm of my hands.

For most of my life, I believed in a world I could only see through my parents' eyes, but not for all of my life. I woke up, looked inside and outside, and then I saw space, and that space connected me to the most healing energy of all: divine wisdom. It came through me and levitated in front of me like that little angel I saw in the window when I was four. There was more truth in what I could not see than in my reality, yet my reality shifted dramatically.

For me, the ruler of the spiritual dimension of health is one I refer to as Spirit, but you can call it whatever you want. You may call it a coincidence or juju, Lord, or Buddha. It is a relationship between yourself and the things you cannot see that is backed by trust, so you can surrender. It means that every spirited action you take is filled with possible outcomes, so many that you cannot wait to see how life will unfold for you. It is an energetic force that dwells inside the cavities of your mind, body, and soul like a soft wind at your back, helping you run swiftly and gracefully upward.

A Spirited Conversation

Power is a product of our human desire to control. Force is a gift that shows us we are out of control by moving us toward less resistance, an invitation to loosen our grip on the bedside and the handlebars—the tug or maybe a jolt that says, "It's right here waiting for you."

I am moved by a life force of energy that helps me clean out my painful body daily. I get to catch the messages, understand the truth being delivered, and embody that truth through spirited acts of authenticity that create a life I live on purpose.

> Work nearly killed me.
> Or I nearly killed myself.
> Paying attention to the guideposts saved me.

I made new agreements with myself, creating a soul plan and contract between Spirit and me. I heal my wounds daily through the cellular death of the things holding me back from a long, purposeful, and healthy life. I get to help others do that, too.

When you are physically ill, it is very hard to stay positive. Some people make it look easy to be perpetually positive, but that is rare. Unblocking my physical, mental, and emotional energy saved my life and healed me into a state of purpose. I began at 46 years old. It wasn't too late. I was right on time. When I was in the waiting room at Johns Hopkins, fighting cancer alone during the pandemic, the work I had done through my mystery illness saved me. Sitting there, I accepted my diagnosis, but I knew that underneath the bald head was a mind that changed the matter of the makeup of what would live and die in my body.

Why was this happening to me?

I am so grateful that after completing chemotherapy in late 2020, Peter Bonaker told me that he thought it was time to go through shamanic training and certification. Like my decision to leave my corporate career, I answered the calling two years later. Cancer was another guidepost that had given me the precursory education I needed to confront death. After I had time to integrate the learnings, I knew I was ready.

I play with my human experience more now, and consider that when new challenges arise, it is a test of my inner guidance system sent from Spirit to help me make the most of my existence. I embrace my nature as a man who loves to drink green juice and appreciates sharing a few glasses of fine wine with friends. There is no Jekyll and Hyde because there are no secrets. I embrace moments of tears and allow them to stream down my face. My long and healthy life is a continuous act of reparenting that nurtures unconditional love and a deep understanding that I am made of many parts.

The "Great Unraveling[IP]" from the fear-based world was once a thing I considered to be a period of the past tense that I now use to heal and connect with divine knowledge. Work is required to communicate with the Spirit. There is no way to bypass our lives. We have to take cues from the existential guideposts and act from an enthusiastic and determined place. We must want it so badly that we are willing to do things differently.

We have all had times when we have felt desperate or broken, pushed to the edge with no one to help us. In those times, we think that Spirit might swoop in and save us if we ask, missing the truth that, more than likely, our struggle is the call to be answered. There's no bypassing the fear-based world. We have to confront it to learn, love, and heal while we are in it before we can transcend it.

There was a time when I didn't notice the lessons in my life because I had labeled them as crappy situations that God was placing on my lap for some unknown reason. My eyes would roll back in sync with my head, and I would say, "What now? Again? Seriously?" as if I had no role to play in the situation.

The man on the plane who lost his wife helped me see that I had other options. The robin knocking on my door informed me that I was on the right track. More and more good and validating information came through as I healed.

Spirit, the Universe, God, and energy live inside us. We are the same. There is no disconnection. Since the start of my Great Unraveling, I have felt closer to Spirit, and it has nothing to do with sitting on a church pew. I'm not telling you to abandon religion. It is a matter of not waiting to enter a building to connect to a higher power. We can get the answers we need to move us into a state of purpose from anywhere at any time.

When we sweep the entrance of our front door, we end the wars and stop trying to make our kingdom larger. If we truly are spiritual beings having a spiritual experience, we must look inside ourselves, draft a peace treaty, and raise the white flag. What would happen if we turned a dream of peace, love, and understanding into a reality of removing the toxic invasion of bad information and false conditioning that is the root cause of external conflicts?

Are You Coming with Me?

You likely have your version of the ride that I took, a time when you struggled repeatedly, but your spirit prevailed. That's what it takes: a commitment to stay with whatever you find. Let's continue to be unafraid to go deep together to fly to the place where profound cellular healing occurs. Let's bring back belly-flexing laughter and newfound connections you can create with your life experiences so you can appreciate every damn second you have lived up until this moment. Let's rewrite our stories to help us heal in the here and now and beyond.

"I don't know what you are doing, but keep on doing what you are doing." My oncologist says this to me every time I go in for a check-up. Yes, I still go to the logical spaces. I get a kick out of sharing the illogical work I do with my medical doctor here in the US. I also travel to Germany to see my integrative doc and continue exploring many illogical spaces.

Accepting that I would never know exactly what treatments and modalities ultimately cured me, I knew one thing for sure: I healed myself. And if a guy like me can heal himself, you can too.

Every day, we can transcend the fear-based world. There's a Rocket Shaman in all of us.[IP] Now it's time to ask you another question.

Are you coming with me?

READER REFLECTION: PREPARING TO LAUNCH YOUR LONG AND HEALTHY LIFE

Looking back on your answers to the questions posed in each chapter of this book, what are your biggest realizations?

What have you learned, and how can you use that learning to heal yourself emotionally, mentally, physically, and spiritually?

Why is it never too late for you to begin the Great Unraveling of your life? How can starting now benefit you tomorrow?

ACTIONABLE INSIGHTS TO HEAL ACROSS FOUR DIMENSIONS OF HEALTH

Emotional

By acknowledging and releasing pain in challenging moments, you can experience the joy of endurance, fostering emotional resilience and growth through adversity.

Mental

Overcoming mental limitations allows you to shift from striving toward external success to embracing the process, leading to fulfillment and clarity in your life's journey.

Physical

Physical endurance and strength are reflections of emotional and mental balance. By healing from within, you restore your health and achieve greater well-being.

Spiritual

Connecting with *Spirit* or a higher power helps you transcend the limits of the physical world, revealing that divine wisdom and guidance can lead to spiritual expansion and purpose.

SPIRITED ACT OF AUTHENTICITY: HOW TO CREATE YOUR PERSONAL VISION BOARD AND MANIFEST YOUR FUTURE

Everything physical is trailing energy. If it hasn't manifested yet, it's just catching up. To shift your reality, you don't change the outside; you recode your field.

The lump came back after chemo. The fear was real: sharp and paralyzing. The doctors had no clear answers. Just more treatments, more uncertainty. It would've been easy to collapse into the story of "I am sick. I am broken." But I refused.

I began with the Identity Shift: "I live a long and healthy life. I am healthy." I repeated the words and declared them as if every cell in my body was listening.

Then came the Emotional Signal. I closed my eyes and felt it. I pictured my healed body walking barefoot on the earth. Laughing. Traveling. Teaching. Breathing with ease. I gave my nervous system a new blueprint. I felt myself whole, vibrant, laughing in the sun, leading others from a place of power and peace. I saw my future. I felt my vitality. I let it rise.

Then I turned to Repetition. I said it in the mirror every morning. I whispered it during moments of doubt. I anchored it into my breath, into my bones: "I live a long and healthy life. I am healthy. I feel my vitality rising. I stabilize this frequency."

This is Activation. This is how I rewrote my reality—not by bypassing the fear but by choosing to speak a deeper truth until my body remembered it too.

Creating a Vision Board is another way to manifest and is one of the most fun tools for activating and anchoring your vision for your future. There are many instructions out there. One of my favorite ones is the one I've learned from Colette Baron-Reid.[38] She divides her Vision Boards into four cornerstones: Intention, Inspiration, Vision, and Action.

I will summarize what I have learned, but I encourage you to book a class with her. She possesses decades of experience manifesting for herself and others.

Intention

- Think about the areas of your life you want to re-infuse with new energy or start anew. The typical areas are

Family/Pets, Love and/or Friendships, Hobbies, Health/ Wellbeing, Job/Calling, Finances, Home Environment, and Philanthropy.

- Now, pick a few and write down your intentions for each. Ideally, you don't pick more than four areas for this step.

Inspiration

- Pick some of your favorite magazines, use Pinterest boards, or search the internet to find pictures that represent your vision for each of the areas you've chosen in the previous step.

  For instance, you dream of a lake house for your home environment. Find a picture that represents your vision of what this should look like. You don't need to find that exact house; you can focus on the feeling you get when you pick a photo of it. This will be important in the next step. You can also pick key phrases such as: "I invite new and exciting adventures into my life."

- Cut these pictures out and save them for later.

Vision

- Purchase a poster board, one that you would use for a school presentation, and start creating your vision. In the center of it, place a picture that represents your picture of *Spirit* or the Divine.

- Separate the vision board into four sections (top left, top right, bottom right, bottom left).

- Next, arrange the pictures you've cut out in the previous step until you feel the board is nicely balanced. Glue them on the vision board.

- Lastly, write "Thank you" several times on and/or around the board's edges. An attitude of gratitude is important in properly manifesting your vision and future.

Action

Now that your vision board is done, it's time to activate it.

- Find a prominent place in your house where you can see your vision board throughout the day.

- Write one or several affirmations about what each section represents. These should be written in the present tense and start with "I am." The simple "trick" to manifesting properly is pretending that what you desire is already so.

- Release any attachments to the outcome and get into the space of feeling. What does it feel like when you sit on the deck of your lake house, sipping coffee? What does it feel like when your bank account always has enough money?

Each day for the next 30 days, I invite you to sit in front of your vision board and get into that feeling state for each category. Colette even suggests biting into a lemon or drinking lemon water to trick the mind into believing that what you're looking at on your board is already reality. I personally like to get into a feeling state and pretend it has already happened. Lately, with the advancement of AI, you can even create images of yourself in that desired situation. I find this super useful for people who otherwise struggle to visualize with their eyes closed.

Have some fun with this. Again, it is more important to be in the feeling than the attachment or "urgent need" state. I love the saying: "This or something better for the benefit of all."

Let the abundance of the Universe surprise and bless you.

Sacred Scribbles *(Use these pages as a portal for decoding visions, tracking soul whispers, or just letting the ink remember what your heart already knows.)*

PART 4. BECOMING THE ROCKET SHAMAN

ACTIVATE YOUR LONG AND HEALTHY LIFE

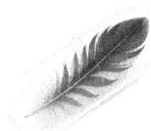

The new caretakers of the Earth will come from the West, and those who have made the greatest impact on Mother Earth now have the moral responsibility to remake their relationship with Her after remaking themselves.

—Don Antonio Morales (Master Q'ero shaman)

For Neo-Shamans, myself included, receiving the **Munay-Ki rites**—a sacred series of energetic transmissions passed down from the Q'ero paqos—is the heartbeat of spiritual initiation. These rites don't simply mark a ceremony; they restructure your energetic or luminous body, installing new architecture that transforms how you perceive and interact with the world. Each transmission plants seeds of ancient wisdom that bloom into specific gifts: the Seer's ability to perceive beyond the veil, the Wisdom Keeper's connection to sacred knowledge, the Earth Keeper's communion with Mother Earth herself. These are commitments woven into the very fabric of our energy field, forever altering our capacity to heal, to serve, and to bridge worlds.

"**Munay-Ki**" means "I love you" or "Be as thou art" in Quechua, the language of the Q'ero. These rites connect us with the ancient wisdom of the **Earthkeepers** and transform and upgrade our energy fields. In shamanic traditions, Earthkeepers are viewed as guardians who connect with and maintain the balance of the Earth, whether as human stewards, spiritual beings, or elements of nature.

It was March 2022 when I first received the Rites. I was driving up to the Berkshires in Massachusetts to complete my certification as an Energy Medicine Practitioner. I can still see the room where I sat with five other apprentices, each of us carrying our own wounds and yearnings. There was Sarah, a yoga teacher whose hands shook with decades of years of generational pain; Denise, recently laid off and searching for meaning; and David, supporting his girlfriend through a profound spiritual awakening. We leaned in, captivated by Peter Bonaker's teachings and the mystery of the Munay-Ki. Peter moved like water between worlds, his presence both grounding and ethereal—a man who'd spent years with the Q'ero and now served as a bridge for seekers like us.

When I say *Rites*, I mean sacred rituals and ceremonies that don't just touch the spirit but rewire it. The Munay-Ki consist of nine powerful energetic transmissions. One of them, called the **Hampe Karpay** (the Earth Keeper's Rite), is the most powerful for me. This wasn't just about becoming a healer—it was about accepting guardianship of the living Earth. The rite awakens dormant codes within your DNA, attuning you to the consciousness of mountains, waters, winds, and fires. Suddenly, you can feel the Earth's joy and pain as if it were your own.

The memory burns bright: a cozy cabin at night, the training drawing to a close, firelight flickering in the log burner, gentle music weaving through the air. But I wasn't prepared for what would come. As we moved to different stations to receive the Rites, my body began to tremble and shake. When Peter placed his hands on my crown for the Hampe Karpay, the energy hit like lightning. My spine became a river of fire. I gasped, doubling over, certain I would vomit or pass out. "Breathe through it," Peter whispered. "Your energy body is reorganizing. Let it."

Then the tears came—not gentle drops but body-shaking sobs. Through the intensity, I felt them: thousands of Earth Keepers throughout time, welcoming me home. The land itself seemed to rise up through the floorboards, embracing me. This wasn't just an initiation; it was a remembering. As if every cell in my body suddenly recalled its purpose. The search for love hadn't ended—it had inverted. I was no longer seeking love; I was becoming a vessel for it to flow through.

At that moment, I understood: the Earth Keeper's path would demand everything. It would require me to feel the Earth's wounds as my own, to stand for healing even when others called me crazy. Perhaps this was the first glimpse of what would later emerge as the "Rocket Shaman"—one who bridges ancient Earth wisdom with cosmic consciousness, grounding stellar frequencies into planetary healing. The Hampe Karpay had given me not just the ability but the responsibility to be this bridge.

10

KNOWING WHAT'S YOURS
TO HEAL

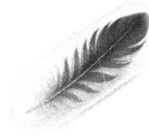

Y ou've reached a pivotal moment in your journey through
this book. It's time to integrate the knowledge, insights,
and lessons. Becoming The Rocket Shaman is not just
a concept; it's a call to reclaim your authentic self, align your
life with your true purpose, and heal emotionally, mentally,
physically, and spiritually.

Many of us go through life on autopilot, shaped by expectations, societal norms, and the desires of others, which create
an internal and external attachment to the fear-based world.
We're born into a reality that has already formed ideas of who
we should be, and without realizing it, we often live out these
scripts rather than writing our own. This can lead to a deep
disconnection from our true selves, leaving us feeling unfulfilled and trapped in lives that don't reflect who we truly are.

As we've explored throughout this book, resetting or healing is about more than just addressing symptoms or finding
temporary relief. It's about going back to the core of your being,
understanding the influences that have shaped you, and choosing the life you want to live. It's about reclaiming your identity
from the forces that have shaped it without your consent, and

rediscovering the child-like voice within you that has always known who you truly are.

The journey of self-love is central to healing. When we misunderstand this concept, we often seek love and acceptance externally, neglecting our needs and worth. We try to fix ourselves when we feel unloved, not realizing that we aren't broken to begin with. We fill our lives with material possessions, achievements, and the approval of others, but these are meaningless without self-love.

Healing is an inherent process within our bodies. Our biological design is a cycle of continuous renewal and regeneration. For instance, the entire lining of our stomach is replaced every few days to keep up with its harsh environment.

The key to understanding this issue lies in our internal and external environments. Internally, our minds may be cluttered with anxiety, negative thoughts, and unprocessed emotions. Externally, we are surrounded by processed foods, harmful chemicals, and a relentless stream of stress and fear from media exposure. These combined forces interfere with our body's natural ability to heal, making it challenging to sustain good health. However, by recognizing these influences and making intentional choices that nurture our body's innate healing powers, we can start to regain balance and restore our vitality.

Remember the concept of circular time used in shamanic healing, traveling back and forth through the past, present, and future? That's a model for how you can use this book. Go back to learning again and again to help you gain new insights into how you can activate on behalf of authenticity to love and heal continuously. Visit the illogical and logical spaces and create your unique approach to designing the long and healthy life you want to live on purpose.

As I write these final chapters, I reflect on the path that led me here and the honor of supporting you in moving through your healing journey. We have been immersed in storytelling throughout *Becoming the Rocket Shaman,* and now, it is time to get out of the story and back into your life. Facing reality isn't as easy as reading a book and theorizing about what we want to have happen. For this reason, I want to give you a tool for moments when no person or thing is there to help you transcend the fear-based world. As you listen to your intuition, allow the existential guideposts to reveal new lessons you can use to transform how you are living your life, decondition yourself to receive the full scope of love that you deserve, and take action to release yourself from your pain body. Your true nature will rise to the surface.

When I finally understood what it meant to live authentically, I stopped feeling like I was juggling multiple lives—working in corporate, exploring my spiritual side, and trying to define my true purpose. For years, I struggled to find the connection between the different roles I played in my life: husband, father, executive, healer, son, and founder. I felt disjointed, as if each aspect of myself was living in a silo. I found that healing happens by aligning ourselves with our one true self that shows up whole and consistent in all areas of our lives. Who we are at our core helps us heal, and healing helps us find who we are at our core.

The truth is that living authentically can be difficult at first, as we face a fear-based world filled with false conditioning and bad information. I hope your experience reading this book and moving through the exercises and Spirited Acts of Authenticity has helped you come to new realizations and take action toward living a long and healthy life. With trial and error, you will realize that you can never go back to a life based on fulfilling the expectations of others or avoiding judgment.

Living authentically gives us the freedom to focus on what truly matters: healing ourselves, serving others, and walking in our purpose. This freedom is the key to not only surviving but thriving in a world that often tries to tell us otherwise. When we live from a place of authenticity, we not only create a more meaningful and fulfilling life for ourselves but also inspire others to do the same, contributing to a healthier, more compassionate world.

By focusing on healing and aligning our lives with our true purpose, we improve our well-being and extend our lives upward and onward. As the antidote to the fear-based world, authenticity, grounded in self-awareness, self-compassion, and purpose, brings a profound sense of peace, which is the foundation of a long, healthy, and meaningful life.

When you live authentically, you transcend the pressures to conform, compete, or survive in ways that don't align with your truth. You no longer make decisions based on fear but from a place of inner peace and purpose. Living a long, healthy life means not being pulled in a thousand directions by others' expectations. Instead, you are grounded, clear, and empowered to live as you choose.

The path to transcending the fear-based world lies in reclaiming what's yours and returning the rest. By sending back the false narratives, unrealistic expectations, and external conditioning, you create the space to heal and live authentically.

What's Yours to Heal vs. What's Not

In our journey through life, much of our baggage doesn't belong to us. It's not always easy to see the difference between what is truly ours to heal and what society, family, and culture have imposed upon us. I hope this helps you practice knowing the difference between what can be returned and what is valuable material to help you heal and create a long, healthy life.

Recognizing What's Yours: The Internal Clues

The first step in healing is to recognize what is truly yours. Your wounds, emotional pain, and unresolved issues will usually manifest as recurring themes in your life. These might show up as

- **Physical symptoms:** Tension, chronic pain, or unexplained illnesses often signal unprocessed emotions or trauma.

- **Emotional patterns:** Feelings of anxiety, guilt, shame, or resentment that repeatedly arise, especially in certain situations or relationships, can be indicators of deeper wounds that need your attention.

- **Mental loops:** Constantly ruminating on a particular fear or belief may suggest a personal block that needs healing.

- **Spiritual disconnection:** Feeling lost, ungrounded, or unsure of your purpose often points to unresolved spiritual questions that require self-reflection.

If these experiences feel profoundly personal and keep showing up, they are likely yours to heal. These are areas where your soul is asking you to grow, evolve, and release what no longer serves you.

Identifying False Conditioning: The External Voices

On the other hand, many of the burdens we carry aren't even ours. They stem from external sources like society's expectations, cultural norms, family pressures, or the voices of authority figures in our lives. These external pressures are based in fear and often manifest in ways that push us to conform, please others, or live up to unrealistic standards. Here's how to recognize them:

PRACTICAL STEPS TO DIFFERENTIATE WHAT'S YOURS VS. WHAT'S NOT

1. **Identify recurring patterns.** Journal about situations that repeatedly cause you pain or discomfort. Are these rooted in your own beliefs, or were they instilled by someone else?

2. **Check the source.** When a belief or emotion comes up, ask yourself, "Whose voice is this? Where did this come from?"

3. **Let go of external validation.** Reflect on decisions you've made recently. Were they to please others or to align with your authentic self?

4. **Suppose you need to process the emotions you are experiencing.** For now, I suggest just journaling about the experience, the person, or force that projected their expectations or fears onto you. Don't judge it or do something about it; we'll get to that later.

By understanding what's truly yours to heal and what belongs to the fear-based world, you can direct your energy toward genuine growth and healing. The result? A lighter, freer, and more empowered version of yourself, unburdened by the weight of the world's expectations.

Now that you've begun to identify what truly belongs to you versus what's been imposed by others, you might be wondering: *What do I actually do with everything that isn't mine?* How do I release these false narratives, expectations, and projections that have been weighing me down for years—maybe even decades?

In the next chapter, I'll share with you a powerful practice I've developed called **Return to Sender.** It's a simple yet profound tool that has freed me from carrying other people's judgments, fears, and expectations. But first, take time to sit with what you've discovered here. The recognition must come before the release. Once you can clearly see what isn't yours, you'll be ready to send it back.

READER REFLECTION: DECIDING WHAT'S YOURS TO HEAL

What emotional, physical, mental, and spiritual patterns have shown up repeatedly in your life that feel personal? What might these signals be trying to teach you about what's truly yours to heal?

Can you recall a belief, expectation, or role you've carried that feels more like a product of someone else's narrative than your own truth? What would it feel like to release it?

If you were to live a life guided only by what is truly yours to heal and express, what parts of your current life would stay, and what would fall away?

ACTIONABLE INSIGHTS TO HEAL ACROSS FOUR DIMENSIONS OF HEALTH

Emotional

By identifying and owning your part in the recurring emotional patterns of your life, you claim what's yours, take responsibility, and release what's not yours to focus on transforming the role you play in your reality into a leader.

Mental

Distinguishing between internal truth and external conditioning clears mental clutter, allowing you to rewrite limiting beliefs with clarity and compassion.

Physical

Letting go of burdens that aren't yours to carry can alleviate chronic tension and restore balance, giving your body space to regenerate and thrive.

Spiritual

Returning false narratives and realigning with your authentic self creates spiritual coherence, helping you reconnect with your purpose and live in greater alignment with your soul's path.

SPIRITED ACT OF AUTHENTICITY: SAND PAINTING RITUAL—RELEASING THE OLD, RECLAIMING THE TRUE

Across traditions—from the high Andes to the Navajo mesas, the Tibetan temples to Aboriginal Dreamtime—people have knelt to the Earth to lay out what cannot be spoken in words. They have shaped grief into feathers, mapped heartbreak with stones, and surrendered old stories to the wind.

The Sand Painting Ritual is one of those sacred acts: an invitation to *externalize the invisible, witness what you're carrying,* and allow *Spirit* and Earth to become active participants in your healing.

This is not about making something pretty. This is about making something *true,* then letting it change.

I've learned this particular process from the Q'ero tradition of the high Andes, an ancient lineage of Earth-honoring shamans. The Q'ero shamans believe that the *sand painting ritual* is a sacred way to externalize inner wounds, stuck energies, outdated stories, or heavy emotions. But unlike art for display, this is impermanent and purposeful. When we build a mandala of meaning with natural materials, we give *Spirit* a map to help us transform the energetic imprints we are ready to release.

I've adapted this sacred work over the years. In this Rocket Shaman work, healing becomes tactile, and truth becomes visible. You create what's ready to be seen, then ceremonially destroy it, inviting Spirit and Earth to complete the energetic process.

The Purpose

- This ritual offers you a symbolic mirror to:
- See what is truly yours to heal and what is not.
- Represent key relationships or events, and where they live in your field.
- Witness how time, nature, and intention begin to move the energy.
- Surrender outcomes to Spirit, and be amazed by what unfolds in your inner and outer life.

What You'll Need:

- A quiet space outdoors or on your balcony/patio
- A cloth or patch of earth for your circle
- Natural objects that *symbolize aspects of your life*:
  - Stones, feathers, twigs, shells, bones, dried flowers, etc.
  - Collect them intentionally—each item representing a *person, a dynamic, an emotion, or a part of your story.*
  - Consider how these relate to one another. Are some close? Some at odds? Do some belong outside your circle?

The Ritual: Step-by-Step

1. Create a Gentle Sacred Space

Stand quietly. Place one hand on your heart and one on your belly. Say aloud or silently:

> "I am stepping into sacred space now. May this be a space of truth, release, and renewal. May I be supported by all that is loving, wise, and unseen."

Feel your body settle. Imagine the Earth rising to meet you.

2. Draw Your Circle

Use twigs, string, or small stones to create a visible circle or rectangular shape on the ground, representing a picture frame. This is your energetic container—your mythic canvas.

3. Place Your Objects with Meaning

One by one, bring in the items you've gathered. With each object, silently or aloud, name what it represents:

*   A person who has shaped you (positively or painfully)
*   An emotion you're ready to transform
*   A dream long buried
*   A version of yourself you're ready to reclaim or release

Place the objects *in relationship* to one another—close or far apart, inside or outside the circle, to reflect the current reality. For example:

*   A painful relationship may sit *outside the circle*, indicating a need for boundaries.
*   A feather placed beside a stone may represent *hope softening heaviness*.

This is not art. This is energetic cartography.

4. Let It Speak

Sit quietly before your painting. Observe what's been revealed. What feels off? What feels right? Don't rush to fix—just *witness*.

> "Words are the language of the mind. Objects are the language of the soul."

Ongoing Integration (7 Days)

Leave your sand painting open and undisturbed for up to a week. Each day:

- Visit it with reverence and curiosity
- Observe how *wind, rain, animals, or light* may have changed the design
- Feel free to move pieces, shift positions, add or remove items based on how your inner world is evolving
- Ask yourself: *How is nature participating in this transformation? What am I feeling in my life that mirrors these shifts?*

This becomes a *daily communion* between your unconscious, the Earth, and *Spirit*.

Completing the Ritual

When you feel the cycle is complete—when the weight has lightened or clarity has arrived—it's time to release the painting.

- Scatter the elements back into nature
- Bury them in the Earth
- Offer them to a fire, river, or ceremonial space
- Or keep one small piece as a reminder of what you've let go

Say aloud:
"I release what is mine to heal. I return what is not mine to carry. I walk forward with clarity, love, and the support of all that is sacred."

Close sacred space by simply placing your hand back on your heart and saying:

"This space is now complete. I am grateful. I am free."

Final Note

Many who perform this ritual report that *their lives begin to shift in subtle and sometimes profound ways* in the days that follow. Emotions move. Conversations open. Dreams return.

Let this be a reminder: healing is not always loud. Sometimes, it begins with a feather in the dirt, a stone on the ground, and your willingness to see clearly what is yours and what never was.

Sacred Scribbles *(Use these pages as a portal for decoding visions, tracking soul whispers, or just letting the ink remember what your heart already knows.)*

11

RETURN TO SENDER

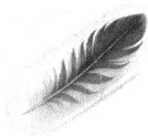

I n the previous chapter, you learned to distinguish between what's truly yours to heal and what belongs to others. Now comes the practical work: actively releasing what isn't yours. The result of understanding what's yours to heal is moving beyond fear-based living. To do that, I've created a very powerful tool called *Return to Sender*. Think of it as the action step that follows your newfound awareness. You've identified the foreign energies, false narratives, and imposed expectations— now it's time to send them back.

The concept sounds simple, but it carries immense weight. In life, we take on the energy, opinions, and judgments of others, whether we realize it or not. Sometimes, that energy can seep into our psyche, making us doubt ourselves, question our path, or feel burdened by the expectations of others. An example in my life was the formation of part of my identity that was constructed from the projections my grandmothers placed on me before I was even born. I've come to understand something important: not everything that comes your way belongs to you. Not everything is yours to heal.

A tangible example that happens often is through communication and conversations in the fear-based world. Think about a time you have received an email, text message, phone call, online review, comment on your social media, or other communication full of criticism, doubt, or negativity. Maybe someone is pointing a finger at you or seems to have an issue with how you are showing up authentically. You have two choices on how to deal with this situation: react or respond (as discussed in Chapter 2). Reacting might look like opening it, reading it, and internalizing everything inside, ruminating, calling five friends to tell them about it, and maybe even sending a message back in defense of yourself. The other way forward would be to respond. A response could look like a well-thought-out reply and an engagement of the other person, but often, I find myself explaining my authentic way of being or becoming, which can lead to energetic distractions. If you are being delivered messages from the fear-based world in reaction to showing up as your whole, incredibly human, and amazing self, there's a way forward that will help you avoid being cornered by judgment or inquisitions of the fear-based world.

After you read the message, mentally, emotionally, and if you so choose, physically, mark it "Return to Sender" and send it right back to them. Being in your authenticity can only transcend the fear-based world when we have methods to avoid getting wrapped up in its chaos. This is a gentle way to hold a mirror up to someone else. In the case of my grandmothers, given that they have transitioned, I compassionately sent them back the boy who was a burden and the child who came to the rescue. "It's no longer mine," I said out loud, and mentally and emotionally allowed the bad information and false conditioning to travel back where it came from. I have also literally returned messages that I have received back to the person who sent them in situations that felt threatening to my authentic self.

One of the most profound moments when I used this practice was when I received some unexpected feedback from a family member after making my work in the healing arts public. His message came over a social media platform, and in all capital letters, he asked me if I had abandoned Jesus because of my work as a Neo-Shaman. The message stung for a moment. In the exclamations, even though he threw a few question marks into the message, there was no sign of curiosity, only animosity and prejudice toward the person he perceived me to have become.

In response, I took a deep breath, closed my eyes, and mentally sent his negativity back to him, not with malice, but with the understanding that his criticism was rooted in his own issues, not mine. But I didn't stop there. I copied his message, and without adding anything to it, I pasted it into a message back to him and pressed send. His discomfort was his, not mine. No longer having to explain who I am is one of the best feelings I have ever felt.

Sending the message back to him, I was no longer tethered to his judgment. I was free.

This simple act is a reminder that you don't have to absorb the energy or opinions of others. You can choose to send it back, to release what doesn't serve you. It's a powerful exercise in protecting your own energy and staying true to who you are. Let them keep their letter. You've got your own path to walk.

It's crucial to understand that **Return to Sender** is not a tool for avoiding accountability or dismissing legitimate concerns in our professional or personal relationships. When someone provides valid feedback about work we've agreed to do, or expresses frustration about unmet commitments, that's not a projection to send back—that's information to consider and respond to thoughtfully. This practice is specifically for releasing false narratives about who you are at your core, not for deflecting responsibility for your actions or agreements. Return to Sender is about spiritual sovereignty, not spiritual bypassing.

All of the labels others use to define you that do not resonate with you, return them to the sender. When you encounter assumptions or ridicule for showing up in alignment with your core values and belief systems, simply return them to the sender. All the directives you are given to follow are safe and right, even though you know they aren't your pathway; return to sender. The freedom you will feel if you practice this consistently will be profound.

It's important to understand that this is not an act of anger or confrontation. It's an act of release and self-love—a way to remind yourself that you don't have to carry someone else's burden, insecurity, or negativity. It is an act of healing because you are committed to not storing the fear-based world in your mind, body, and soul. It's an act of self-preservation and peace.

The fear-based world is rooted in ideas of lack, competition, and unworthiness. It convinces us that we must always strive for more success, more validation, and more security because who we are, as we are, isn't enough. This constant striving pulls us away from our true selves and leaves us feeling disconnected from our purpose. The more we cling to these external narratives, the more fragmented and unnatural our identities become.

When we live authentically, we cultivate an inner peace that promotes physical, mental, and emotional well-being.

- **Reduced stress:** Authentic living reduces the stress that comes from trying to meet external expectations. We stop trying to fit into societal boxes and instead, embrace the freedom of being ourselves.

- **Improved health:** The reduction of stress allows our bodies to heal and function optimally. With less anxiety and emotional turmoil, we experience better sleep, a stronger immune system, and more energy.

- **Longevity:** Decades of research show that people who live with a clear sense of purpose and inner alignment not only report greater well-being, but they live longer, healthier lives. Purpose is associated with lower inflammation, stronger immunity, and a significantly reduced risk of disease and early death. When we are connected to our true purpose and living authentically, we experience greater overall satisfaction with life, which contributes to long-term health.

Ultimately, returning the fear-based world's narratives back to sender allows us to reclaim our power. We transcend the need to conform, to please, or to live according to someone else's script. Instead, we embrace our own path, one that aligns with our values, our desires, and our unique purpose.

READER REFLECTION: UNSUBSCRIBING FROM LABELS, LIES, AND LEGACIES THAT AREN'T YOURS

What messages, labels, or projections have you been carrying that were never yours to hold? Can you name one and intentionally practice sending it back with compassion?

When was the last time someone's judgment or fear-based communication made you question your path? What would it feel like to mark it "Return to Sender" instead of internalizing it?

How might your physical, emotional, or spiritual health change if you consistently released the weight of what isn't yours to heal? What becomes possible when you choose peace over explanation?

ACTIONABLE INSIGHTS TO HEAL ACROSS FOUR DIMENSIONS OF HEALTH

Emotional

Sending back what isn't yours helps you release feelings of guilt, shame, and unworthiness that don't belong to you. This allows you to focus on your authentic emotional needs and heal in a way that nourishes your soul.

Mental

When you stop holding onto false beliefs and conditioning, you free your mind from the clutter of fear-based narratives. This mental clarity allows you to focus on your own thoughts, desires, and truths.

Physical

Your body often stores unhealed emotional and mental pain. By releasing what isn't yours, you may find relief from physical ailments that were a manifestation of carrying others' burdens.

Spiritual

Spiritually, sending back what's not yours creates space for your true self to emerge. You reconnect with your inner purpose, unburdened by the need to conform to others' expectations.

SPIRITED ACT OF AUTHENTICITY: ENERGETIC SOVEREIGNTY RITUAL[IP]—RELEASING WHAT WAS NEVER YOURS

At birth, you were whole. Then came the projections, opinions, judgments, and expectations. You absorbed your parents' fears, your culture's narratives, and society's roles. Some came as praise, others as poison. Either way. They stuck.

As time passes, you begin to carry stories that were never yours to begin with:

"You're too sensitive."

"You'll never be enough."

"You are responsible for my pain."

This ritual is your sacred act of energetic return—a boundary, a declaration, a rebalancing of power. It is not done in hate or anger, but with clarity, love, and spiritual sovereignty.

You are not rejecting people. You are rejecting distortion.[IP] And in doing so, you reclaim the frequency of your truth.

A Brief Historical and Psychological Frame

Throughout cultures and healing traditions, the practice of energetic disentanglement has long been revered:

- In Tibetan Vajrayana Buddhism, advanced practitioners engage in Chöd ceremonies, such as symbolic offerings of their body and identity to sever attachment to ego and inherited fear.

- Huna shamans of Hawaii perform ho'oponopono rituals to cleanse spiritual misalignments and return responsibility to its origin.

- Psychodrama therapy in modern psychology has patients physically role-play inherited scripts and hand back psychic burdens to their "rightful owners."

- In quantum energy fields, we now understand that thought forms and emotional residues can linger in our auric field, disrupting clarity and coherence until consciously discharged.

Modern science has shown that trauma, shame, and limiting beliefs can be epigenetically inherited and energetically mirrored in interpersonal dynamics.[39]

The Purpose of This Ritual

This ritual helps you:

- Cut cords of energetic entanglement and projection
- Identify inherited or imposed beliefs and emotional burdens
- Return those energies with compassion, not confrontation
- Reclaim your space as sacred, sovereign, and whole

What You'll Need:

- A quiet space
- A piece of string, scarf, or cord
- A pair of scissors
- A candle or incense (optional)
- A journal
- Optional: an object that symbolizes the projection (e.g., a stone, a photo, a note)

The Ritual: Step-by-Step

1. Ground and Set Intention

Sit quietly. Place one hand on your chest and one on your belly. Feel your breath.

> Say aloud:
> "I call back my energy from all places where it does not belong. I prepare to return what is not mine to carry."

Imagine a golden light around you; a boundary of loving protection.

2. Name What You're Releasing

In your journal, write down the energies you've absorbed that feel foreign or heavy.

- "I am responsible for someone else's happiness."
- "My body must look a certain way to be lovable."
- "I must shrink to be safe."

Then ask yourself:

- Where did this come from?
- Whose voice is this really?
- Who benefits from me believing this?

3. Create the Cord

Hold the string in both hands. Imagine one end connected to you and the other to the person, belief, or energy you're returning.

Say:
"With compassion, I return this to its source. It is not mine to hold."

Feel into the weight of it. Then cut or untie the cord physically or symbolically.

Breathe deeply. Let the release be real.

4. Use Your Voice (Optional but Powerful)

Speak aloud the projections you are sending back.

- "You are not my voice."
- "I am no longer a mirror for your pain."
- "With love, I return your story to you."

This is not rage. It's resonance.
You may also write a letter that begins:

"These were never mine…"

Then burn it or bury it as a final act of closure.

5. Cleanse Your Field

Light incense or wave your hands around your body with a spritz of Agua de Florida. Say:

"I cleanse my field of all projections, judgments, cords, and expectations that are not mine."

Visualize any lingering attachments dissolving like smoke.

6. Seal with Sovereignty

Place your hand on your heart and say:

> "I belong to myself. I am not a container for others' fears. I live as a sovereign being."

Imagine a protective aura forming around your body—golden, strong, loving.

Aftercare + Observation

This ritual can ripple through your life in mysterious ways.

- You may notice conversations shifting.
- You might suddenly stop taking things personally.
- Physical symptoms may lessen.
- Creative clarity may flood in.

    Just like the sand painting, what you remove in energy can move mountains in matter.

Revisit this ritual any time you feel energetically "invaded" or notice old patterns surfacing.

Energetic sovereignty is not isolation. It is communion through clarity. You were never meant to carry the whole world—only your truth.

Let this ritual be the line in the sand. The gentle "no more." The whisper that says:

> "I remember who I am."

Sacred Scribbles *(Use these pages as a portal for decoding visions, tracking soul whispers, or just letting the ink remember what your heart already knows.)*

CONCLUSION

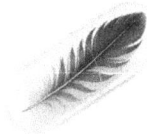

Healthy citizens are the greatest asset any country can have.

—Winston Churchill

Writing this book, I am even more convinced of the healing power of words. Through finding the narratives I wanted to share and processing them repeatedly through the editing process, I found myself on another surprising healing journey. I spilled my guts to the people who helped me write this debut book.

Authorship is ultimately a public exercise in vulnerability, courage, and self-expression, but it has also been a private and personal creative exploration of my existence. The process has strengthened me: mind, body, and spirit. In celebration of my storytelling journey and in anticipation of yours, I invite you to say these words to yourself in the mirror every morning after you rise out of bed. Together, if we change the way we speak about healthcare, perhaps we can change the way we think about it. If that happens, the sky's the limit for what we can do about it.

"I live a life of my design that takes my mind, body, and spirit as high as a rocket can fly. I am healthy."

As I bring this book to a close, I want to leave you with this: no matter how fragmented your life or career might feel right now, there is always a way to bring it all together. The key is alignment—not just in your work, but in your identity. For me, that alignment came through recognizing that I am not just a healer, or a speaker, or an author, or a founder. I am all of those things, and they are all integral parts of who I am. I don't have to play a part or dress a certain way. All I have to do is be myself—the more I get to know him, the more I appreciate the full scope of who I am.

It's taken me years to find this alignment, but now that I have, everything feels clearer and more purposeful. As you navigate your own path, I want to encourage you to embrace all the different aspects of yourself. Don't try to fit into one box. Instead, create your own framework—one that allows all parts of you to thrive.

Thank you for sharing this journey with me. I hope my story has inspired you to find your own alignment, your unique way of showing up in the world. Remember, the parts of your identity aren't in competition. They can coexist harmoniously, creating a rich, fulfilling, and significant life.

YOU'VE FINISHED THE BOOK - NOW LET'S BEGIN THE JOURNEY.

Step fully into the life you're meant to live.

JOIN THE ROCKET SHAMAN CHAT PATHWAY:

CONNECT

HEAL

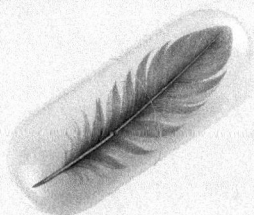

ALIGN

TRANSFORM

APPENDIX A

ENERGETIC ROCKET FUEL[IP]: USING FOOD AND DRINK AS MEDICINE

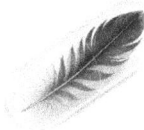

When I was first diagnosed with my autoimmune disease, I knew I had to clean up my diet. Having been born and raised in Switzerland, our breakfast (and dinners) consisted of an array of whole-grain breads, butter, jams, honey, yogurt, and cheeses. While none of those foods are unhealthy, my American lifestyle (driving more, walking less, and less easy access to the highest quality foods), mixed with the inflammation I was experiencing in my body, called me to change the way I nourish my body.

I gave up bread for a lengthy period. You can imagine what it felt like, given that bread had been an important staple of my diet for over forty years. But I can attest to how beneficial it was to simplify my diet, starting with breakfast, to include more plants. Replacing my grain-heavy breakfast with green smoothies helped me reduce water retention, improve digestion, and boost my energy. On top of that, the green smoothies I make are delicious. I crave one shortly after I wake up. While I have integrated an occasional breakfast inspired by those

Sundays with my family back into my life, more often, I would rather have a produce-rich morning.

I chose to go plant-based, gluten and dairy-free for a few years, which I believe to be the key to healing my entire body throughout the years when I was sick. Because I eliminated many types of food, and had a pretty serious reason to do it, I consider it one of the main reasons my integrative doc in Germany pronounced me free from the toxins and food allergies that caused my autoimmune condition. I believe that many of the autoimmune dis-eases and chronic conditions we have today are treatable. It's difficult to get a diagnosis when there's not a lot known about many autoimmune and rare diseases. Using food as medicine helped me choose foods that were healthier for me.

Given the way healthcare is run in the US, it takes patience, perseverance, and, unfortunately, quite a bit of money to confront our personal health, especially when we get sick. Detox services like the one I completed in Germany—though now becoming available in the US—are rarely covered by insurance. Most Western doctors are unaware of the lab tests available for heavy metals and pesticide poisoning in the US, which is why I often felt like they thought I was nuts when I would ask about alternative treatments.

When I was diagnosed in 2016, none of those tests were available to me, and I had to travel to Europe for treatment. The good news is that we're progressing in integrative healthcare, and many fantastic medical doctors are now more equipped and dedicated to providing holistic treatment plans. The bad news is that most of those services require someone to pay out of pocket, which means, unfortunately, these services are out of reach for many. Healthcare equality is a long way away. Hence, I've dedicated my life to changing how we think about healthcare in the Western world. My aim is to raise awareness among people, so that it becomes easier for them to access alternative healing pathways.

In the meantime, there are easy ways to stay healthy or improve your health. I found that, despite being expensive, food costs are more affordable than prescription medication and unexpected medical bills. Starting with viewing food as medicine has been a game-changer for me. With that, I beg you to ditch those sugary drinks you are drinking (if you are drinking them), examine the types and the amount of overly-processed food you are consuming, and revert to healthy fats (in moderation) versus fast-food burgers and fries. Nutrition is a complex subject because every single one of us responds differently to different foods. There is no one-size-fits-all nutrition plan, so I hope by sharing my approach, you might be inspired to create a new way of nourishing your body that will support your long and healthy life. There is emerging research that suggests that a calorie-poor, nutrient-rich, plant-based diet is the way to go, so that's the route I took.

I do not go hungry, and I don't do diets. My focus is on lifestyle change and mindset. When I discovered that Tom Brady and Rich Roll, two top-performing athletes, were on plant-based diets, I no longer worried about lacking energy. While I have stuck to a heavily plant-based diet (about 80 percent of the time), I did add some lean animal protein back into my diet (think grass-fed beef and happy chickens that were free to roam, or wild-caught salmon) a few times per week.

One of my good friends happens to be a pastry chef *and* a health coach. She has given me some great advice, including the recommendation to treat myself to a dessert I love once or twice per month. What initially sounded like a complete contradiction has become an inspiring way for me to build a sustainable and healthy connection with food. Her advice has been that keeping in mind portion management is important and that your attitude towards what you're eating is a way to support a more mindful and satisfying approach to eating. I no longer eat if I think something is bad for me or if I don't like something.

If you're eating with an attitude that your cells are being fueled and that it is good for you, then the idea is that it changes the energy of that food. This doesn't mean to go gorge on potato chips. It means you might decide not to binge and take your time, appreciating them without guiltily shoving them into your mouth. Try it out, play with it, and see how your body responds.

To stretch myself to be adventurous, especially with produce, I ignore the inner aisles of the supermarket where so many processed foods are located, and roam the outer sections where the fresh stuff lives. One of my favorite pleasures is going to the farmers' market and getting ideas from the vendors and inspiration by buying what's in season. I taste more intense flavor in farm-fresh whole foods. I challenge you to bite into a carrot picked that day and see how different it tastes versus one that has been produced in massive quantities, traveled for thousands of miles, and stored for long periods in a plastic bag. Eating fresh vegetables out of his grandmother's garden is what inspired renowned chef Daniel Humm to become a culinary arts expert and ultimately transfer one of the top restaurants in the world, Eleven Madison Park in NYC, to a purely plant-based experience. Even more impressive, he retained the restaurant's 3 Michelin Stars and proved all skeptics wrong.

Because treating food as medicine has made such a positive difference in my life, I am sharing a few of my favorite recipes with you. Some of them are my creations, and others are inspired by culinary professionals and doctors. The recipes are available for download at TheRocketShaman.com/subscribe or by scanning this QR code.

P.S.: Don't forget to buy organic if your wallet allows, and thoroughly wash your produce (even with a skin or peel like oranges and avocados) to remove most of the pesticides if you choose to eat non-organic fruits and vegetables.

Here's to good health, activating your personalized food-as-medicine journey, and launching your longevity rocket.

Simon

APPENDIX B
RESOURCES

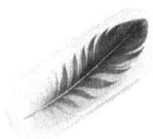

PART 1 RESOURCES: TAKE YOURSELF HIGHER

Masters of the Living Energy: The Mystical World of the Q'ero of Peru
by John Parisi Wilcox

The Four Winds Society
thefourwinds.com

Peter Bonaker, PhD - Shaman, Author, Speaker, Shamanic Teacher
peterbonaker.com

Dreaming With the Wheel: How to Interpret Your Dreams Using the Medicine Wheel
by Sun Bear, Wabun Wind, and Shawnodese

PART 2 RESOURCES: TAKE YOURSELF HIGHER

Mating in Captivity: Unlocking Erotic Intelligence
by Esther Perel

Energy Strands: The Ultimate Guide to Clearing the Cords that Are Constricting Your Life
by Denise Linn

Sacred Shield: Shamanic Protection for the World Today
by Peter Bonaker

Letting Go: The Pathway of Surrender
by David R. Hawkins

On Death and Dying
by Elisabeth Kübler-Ross

You Can Heal Your Life
by Louis Hay

Grow a New Body: How Spirit and Power Plant Nutrients Can Transform Your Health
by Dr. Alberto Villoldo

Grandmothers' Wisdom: Living Portrayals from the International Council of Thirteen Indigenous Grandmothers

PART 3 RESOURCES: TAKE YOURSELF HIGHER

A New Earth: Awakening Your Life's Purpose
by Eckhart Tolle

The Essential Law of Attraction Collection
by Esther and Jerry Hicks

You Can Heal Your Body
by Louise Hay

Shaman, Healer, Sage: How to Heal Yourself and Others with the Energy Medicine of the Americas
by Alberto Villoldo

Life, Love and Transition: Guidance for the End of Life
by Ms Suzanne O'Brien, RN

ENDNOTES

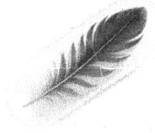

1   Muriel T. Zaatar, Kenda Alhakim, Mohammad Enayeh, and Ribal Tamer, "The Transformative Power of Music: Insights into Neuroplasticity, Health, and Disease," *Brain, Behavior, & Immunity – Health* 35 (2023): article 100716 (e-collection Feb. 2024), doi:10.1016/j.bbih.2023.100716, PMCID PMC10765015.

2   Jagbir Singh, "Prophecies of the Q'ero Inca Shamans," Shri Adi Shakti: The mother goddess, 2024, https://www.adishakti.org/_/prophecies_of_the_qero_inca_shamans.htm.

3   "Q'ero Shamans." *Eomega.org*, 2024. https://www.eomega.org/workshops/teachers/qero-shamans.

4   Parenting Services, "Why Does My Kid Always Ask 'Why'?," Sanford Health News, November 28, 2022, https://news.sanfordhealth.org/parenting/why-does-my-kid-always-ask-why/.

5   Albert R. Broccoli, *Chitty Chitty Bang Bang*, film (20th Century Fox, 1968).

6   Julie Corliss, "Under Pressure: How Stress May Affect Your Heart," Harvard Health, March 1, 2022, https://www.health.harvard.edu/heart-health/under-pressur

e-how-stress-may-affect-your-heart.; "5 Stress Busters
to Help Your Heart," Harvard Health, April 17, 2025,
https://www.health.harvard.edu/heart-health/5-stre
ss-busters-to-help-your-heart.; Huan Song et al., "Stress
Related Disorders and Risk of Cardiovascular Disease:
Population Based, Sibling Controlled Cohort Study,"
BMJ, April 10, 2019, l1255, https://doi.org/10.1136/bmj.
l1255.; "About the CDC-Kaiser Ace Study |Violence
Prevention|injury Center|CDC," Centers for Disease
Control and Prevention, April 6, 2021, https://www.cdc.
gov/violenceprevention/aces/about.html.; Shanta R. Dube
et al., "Cumulative Childhood Stress and Autoimmune
Diseases in Adults," *Psychosomatic Medicine* 71, no.
2 (February 2009): 243–50, https://doi.org/10.1097/
psy.0b013e3181907888.; Carolyn Serraino, "Stress
& Autoimmune Disease: Navigating the Complex
Relationship "Global Autoimmune Institute," Global
Autoimmune Institute", June 3, 2024, https://www.
autoimmuneinstitute.org/articles/stress-autoimmun
e-disease-navigating-the-complex-relationship/.;
"Uncovering the Link between Emotional Stress and
Heart Disease," Harvard Health, April 1, 2017, https://
www.health.harvard.edu/newsletter_article/uncoverin
g-the-link-between-emotional-stress-and-heart-disease.;
"Psychoneuroimmunology," Wikipedia, May 25, 2025,
https://en.wikipedia.org/wiki/Psychoneuroimmunology.

7   *The Lion King*, directed by Roger Allers and Rob Minkoff
     (United States: Buena Vista Pictures, Walt Disney Home
     Video, 1994), film.

8   "The Teen Brain: 7 Things to Know." *National Institute
     of Mental Health*, U.S. Department of Health and
     Human Services, www.nimh.nih.gov/health/publications/
     the-teen-brain-7-things-to-know. Accessed 14 Sept. 2024.

9   What Is Highway Hypnosis and How to Avoid
    It," Cleveland Clinic, June 9, 2023, https://health.
    clevelandclinic.org/highway-hypnosis.

10 Shawnodese, Wabun Wind, and Sun Bear, *Dreaming
    with the Wheel: How to Interpret Your Dreams Using the
    Medicine Wheel* (New York, NY: Touchstone, 2014).

11 Hooper, Lee V., et al. "How Host-Microbial Interactions
    Shape the Nutrient Environment of the Mammalian
    Intestine." *Cell Host & Microbe*, vol. 10, no. 4,
    2011, pp. 297-310. *National Center for Biotechnology
    Information*, https://www.ncbi.nlm.nih.gov/pmc/articles/
    PMC3218761/. Accessed 14 Sept. 2024.

12 Ethan Kross et al., "Social Rejection Shares
    Somatosensory Representations with Physical Pain,"
    Proceedings of the National Academy of Sciences 108, no.
    15 (March 28, 2011): 6270–75, https://doi.org/10.1073/
    pnas.1102693108.

13 Morgan Mandriota, "Lovesick: Yes, It's a Thing," Psych
    Central, October 18, 2021, https://psychcentral.com/
    health/what-is-love-sick.

14 Janice K. Kiecolt-Glaser and Stephanie J. Wilson,
    "Lovesick: How Couples' Relationships Influence
    Health," *Annual Review of Clinical Psychology* 13, no.
    1 (May 8, 2017): 421–43, https://doi.org/10.1146/
    annurev-clinpsy-032816-045111.

15 Denise Linn, *Energy Strands: The Ultimate Guide
    to Clearing the Cords That Are Constricting Your Life*
    (Carlsbad, CA: Hay House, Inc, 2018).

16 Peter Bonaker, *Sacred Shield: shamanic Protection for the
    World Today* (Peter Bonaker, 2020).

17 Low and high vibe response systems are inspired by
    The Map of Consciousness®, a proven energy scale
    to actualize your full potential by M.D., Ph.D.,
    internationally renowned spiritual teacher, psychiatrist,
    physician, researcher, and lecturer David R. Hawkins.

18 "History of Chelation." *AG Patel MD*, www.agpatelmd.
    com/history-of-chelation.html. Accessed 19 Sept. 2024.

19 "Alberto Villoldo – Biography," The Four Winds,
    August 25, 2021, https://thefourwinds.com/
    alberto-villoldo-biography/.

20 Alberto Villoldo, "Grow a New Body: One Week of
    Healing, Renewal and Wisdom," Menla, March 31,
    2024, https://menla.org/retreat/grow-a-new-body-one-wee
    k-of-healing-renewal-and-wisdom/.

21 TM Srinivasan, "Energy Medicine," *International
    Journal of Yoga* 3, no. 1 (2010): 1, https://doi.
    org/10.4103/0973-6131.66770.

22 Wenliang Lv, "Understanding Traditional Chinese
    Medicine," *Hepatobiliary Surgery and Nutrition* 10, no.
    6 (December 2021): 846–48, https://doi.org/10.21037/
    hbsn-2021-25.

23 "How You Can Help Your Baby Build a Better Brain,"
    University Hospitals, February 5, 2018, https://www.
    uhhospitals.org/blog/articles/2018/02/90-percent-of-brain
    -development-occurs-in-first-2000-days.

24 Louise Hay, "Daily Affirmations & Positive Quotes from
    Louise Hay," Louise Hay, May 25, 2017, https://www.
    louisehay.com/affirmations/.

25 "Grandmothers Wisdom Project," GRANDMOTHERS
    WISDOM, accessed September 20, 2024, http://www.
    grandmotherswisdom.org/.

26 "The Great Alaska Shakeout." *Great ShakeOut Earthquake Drills - Select Your ShakeOut Region*, www.shakeout.org/alaska/whyparticipate/index.html#:~:text=EARTHQUAKE%20HAZARDS,move%20relative%20to%20each%20other. Accessed 21 Sept. 2024.

27 *Protective Actions Research*, community.fema.gov/ProtectiveActions/s/article/Earthquake-Personal-Cover-Barriers-Do-Not-Use-a-Doorway#:~:text=Do%20not%20use%20a%20doorway%20except%20if%20you%20know%20it,and%20do%20not%20offer%20protection. Accessed 21 Sept. 2024.

28 Louise L. Hay, *Mirror Work: 21 Days to Heal Your Life* (Carlsbad, CA: Hay House, Inc, 2016).

29 "International End of Life Doula Association." *INELDA*, 10 Apr. 2023, inelda.org/.

30 The Shaman's Universe | Green Tara College." 2019. Greentara.ie. 2019. https://www.greentara.ie/what-is-shamanism/the-shamans-universe.

31 Eckhart Tolle, *A New Earth: Awakening to Your Life's Purpose* (New York, NY: Penguin Books, 2016).

32 Anne Stankewitz et al., *Migraine Attacks as a Result of Hypothalamic Loss of Control*, November 20, 2020, https://doi.org/10.1101/2020.11.19.390104.

33 Lauri Nummenmaa et al., "Bodily Maps of Emotions," *Proceedings of the National Academy of Sciences* 111, no. 2 (December 30, 2013): 646–51, https://doi.org/10.1073/pnas.1321664111.

34 Disease," *Encyclopædia Britannica*, last updated July 18, 2025, edited by The Editors of *Encyclopædia Britannica*, https://www.britannica.com/science/disease.

35 Louise L. Hay, *Heal Your Body: The Mental Causes for Physical Illness and the Metaphysical Way to Overcome Them* (Carlsbad, CA: Hay House, 2012).

36 Alberto Villoldo, Shaman, Healer, Sage: How to Heal Yourself and Others with the Energy Medicine of the Americas (New York, NY: Harmony Books, 2000).

37 "End-of-Life Care Education," Doulagivers, accessed September 20, 2024, https://doulagivers.com/.

38 Colette Baron-Reid, "Vision Board Archives - Colette Baron-Reid: Oracle Cards: Founder of Oracle School," January 2, 2024, https://www.colettebaronreid.com/blog/category/vision-board/.

39 Bruce H. Lipton, *The Biology of Belief: Unleashing the Power of Consciousness, Matter & Miracles* (Carlsbad, CA: Hay House, Inc, 2016).

ACKNOWLEDGMENTS

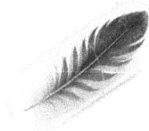

I never thought I'd write a book like this. But after being invited to contribute to a book anthology alongside thirty other authors in late 2023, I realized my stories were worth telling. I want to thank Dr. Taryn Marie Stejskal for inspiring me to participate in the bestselling book *Triumphs of Transformation*, a collection of resilience stories that catalyzed this book. Writing this book has been a deeply healing journey. When I began exploring the root cause of my illness in 2015, I had no idea it would spark a complete life transformation, bring new connections, and help me develop invaluable skills. There is an ancient saying: *"When the student is ready, the teacher will appear."* And so it was.

I want to express my heartfelt gratitude to Dr. Alberto Villoldo, a pioneer in neo-shamanism, for sharing the wisdom of the Q'ero people through his many books. His organization, the Four Winds Society, and his program *Grow a New Body* have profoundly influenced my journey toward living a long and healthy life. I also wish to acknowledge my brother, Valentin, a trailblazer in energy medicine, mediumship, and shamanism, whose example has inspired me to walk this path. A special thanks to Grandmother Rita Pitka Blumenstein for "seeing" and believing in me, and Peter Bonaker, Ph.D., for sharing his teachings and friendship over the years.

I honor my many teachers—Nadine Reuter, Madeleine Andersen, Lisa Saylan, Suzanne O'Brien, Cyndy Paige, Tikirau Ata, Heidi Hüber, and Richard Knight—for their wisdom and guidance.

I want to express my deepest gratitude to the souls who appeared on my path at precisely the right moments, each a divine messenger in human form. To Jeff Pruitt, thank you for planting the seed that would forever change my path; your suggestion to explore Reiki opened a gateway to energy healing that would eventually become the foundation of my life's work. To Ed Borromeo and Daniel Srdic, who reached out when I was navigating the shadows of divorce and loss, thank you for reminding me of my aliveness. Your encouragement to take classes and dream of a new life lit the first candle of hope during my darkest hours. And to Patrick O'Halleran, who saw something in me early in my career. Thank you for holding that vision with such steadfast friendship and belief. Your support over the years has been a quiet but powerful current, helping me rise when I doubted my own wings.

Thank you also to my beta readers—Nicole Miller, Karen Berdoulay, Marleta Ross, Mike Buccialia, George Simpson, Christina Woronchak, Brooke Evans, Ethan Saikin, and Jill Asfoor—for providing invaluable feedback that made this book stronger. Your insights and gentle critiques were instrumental in shaping this manuscript.

A heartfelt thank you to the entire team at Igniting Souls Publishing Agency for supporting me in the final stages of this journey. Your care, expertise, and belief in this message helped bring this book to life with clarity and purpose.

Finally, I bow in reverence to the many Indigenous wisdom keepers—past, present, and future—whose ancestral teachings, earth-honoring ways, and spiritual stewardship have shaped the path I now walk. May this book be a respectful offering in the great circle of remembrance, healing, and reconnection.

Your wisdom and dedication to creating healthy communities and stewarding the land have been a gift, guiding me to find health in both logical and illogical places.

With deep *Munay*,
Simon Lüthi
July 2025

ABOUT THE AUTHOR

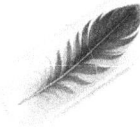

Simon Lüthi, *The Rocket Shaman*, transcended autoimmune disease and cancer by embracing diverse healing methods beyond Western medicine. Leaving the C-Suite, he became a Certified Energy Medicine Practitioner, Reiki Master, Certified End of Life Doula, and the creator of Transmutation Design^{IP}—a new way of working and living that helps conscious leaders feel better, embody presence, and create environments where thriving becomes natural."Leaving his desk on Wall Street to train under the Q'ero Shamans of Peru and a Yup'ik Elder in Alaska, Simon now dedicates his life to reshaping how Americans think about healthcare.

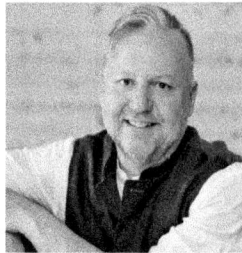

Join Simon on his socials
IG: @therocketshaman
TikTok: @therocketshaman
LinkedIn: linkedin.com/in/simonluthi

Sign up for "The Rocket Shaman," Simon's official newsletter, and get a free gift of his "Rocket Shaman Recipes" e-book.

On his website: TheRocketShaman.com/subscribe

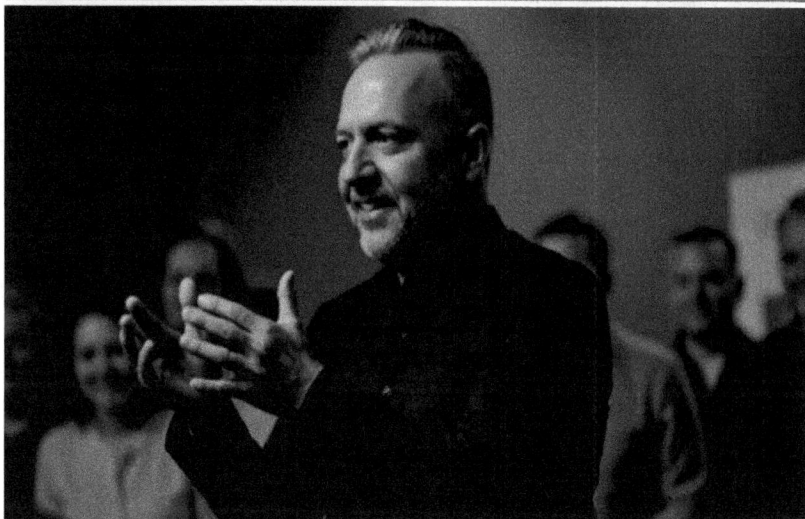

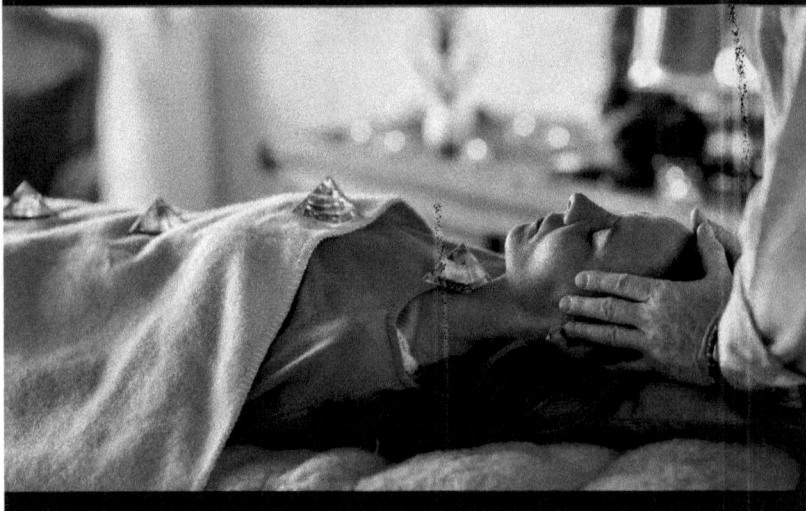

ALIGN
WITH PURPOSE

Stop Living Someone Else's Story

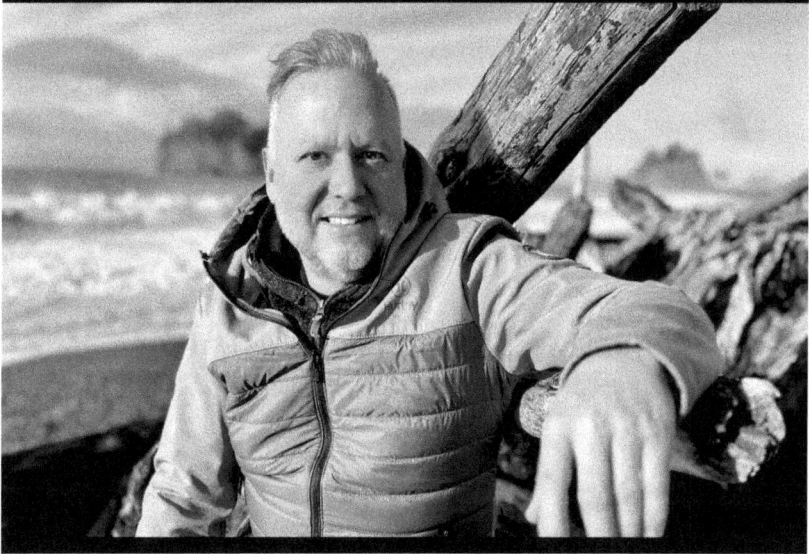

LEARN NOT JUST TO SURVIVE, BUT TO THRIVE.

Rewrite your story, break free from conditioning, and manifest your best life.

Begin Your Hero's Journey Today:
TheRocketShaman.com/Align

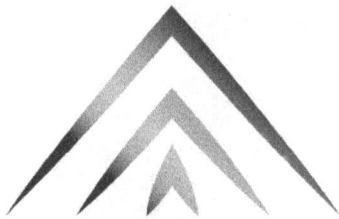

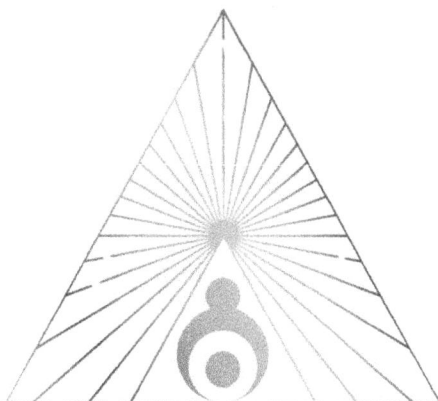

Inner Circle

LIVE TRANSMISSIONS. SACRED RITUALS. A COMMUNITY THAT SEES YOU. GO DEEPER AND TRANSFORM WITH US.

Become A Member

TheRocketShaman.com/InnerCircle

THIS BOOK IS PROTECTED INTELLECTUAL PROPERTY

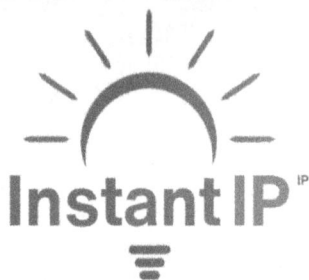

Instant IP [IP]

The author of this book values Intellectual Property. The book you just read is protected by Instant IP[IP], a proprietary process, which integrates blockchain technology giving Intellectual Property "Global Protection." By creating a "Time-Stamped" smart contract that can never be tampered with or changed, we establish "First Use" that tracks back to the author.

Instant IP [IP] functions much like a Pre-Patent since it provides an immutable "First Use" of the Intellectual Property. This is achieved through our proprietary process of leveraging blockchain technology and smart contracts. As a result, proving "First Use" is simple through a global and verifiable smart contract. By protecting intellectual property with blockchain technology and smart contracts, we establish a "First to File" event.

Protected by Instant IP [IP]

LEARN MORE AT INSTANTIP.TODAY